Gestational Diabetes
What to Expect

Fifth Edition

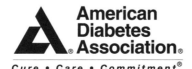

American Diabetes Association®
Cure • Care • Commitment®

Director, Book Publishing, John Fedor; *Managing Editor,* Abe Ogden; *Book Acquisitions,* Sherrye Landrum; *Editor, 5th Edition,* Rebecca Lanning; *Production Manager,* Melissa Sprott; *Cover Design,* Koncept, Inc.; *Printer,* Worzalla Publishing.

Printed in the United States of America
1 3 5 7 9 10 8 6 4 2

The suggestions and information contained in this publication are generally consistent with the *Clinical Practice Recommendations* and other policies of the American Diabetes Association, but they do not represent the policy or position of the Association or any of its boards or committees. Reasonable steps have been taken to ensure the accuracy of the information presented. However, the American Diabetes Association cannot ensure the safety or efficacy of any product or service described in this publication. Individuals are advised to consult a physician or other appropriate health care professional before undertaking any diet or exercise program or taking any medication referred to in this publication. Professionals must use and apply their own professional judgment, experience, and training and should not rely solely on the information contained in this publication before prescribing any diet, exercise, or medication. The American Diabetes Association—its officers, directors, employees, volunteers, and members—assumes no responsibility or liability for personal or other injury, loss, or damage that may result from the suggestions or information in this publication.

♾ The paper in this publication meets the requirements of the ANSI Standard Z39.48-1992 (permanence of paper).

ADA titles may be purchased for business or promotional use or for special sales. To purchase this book in large quantities, or for custom editions of this book with your logo, contact Lee Romano Sequeira, Special Sales & Promotions, at the address below or at LRomano@diabetes.org or 703-299-2046.

American Diabetes Association
1701 North Beauregard Street
Alexandria, Virginia 22311

Library of Congress Cataloging-in-Publication Data

Gestational diabetes : what to expect / American Diabetes Association.-- 5th ed.
    p. cm.
  Includes bibliographical references and index.
  ISBN 1-58040-233-X (alk. paper)
  1. Diabetes in pregnancy--Popular works. I. American Diabetes Association.

RG580.D5G476 2005
618.3--dc22
                              2005026513

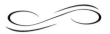

Contents

Acknowledgments

The first edition of this book was written by the Task Force on Gestational Diabetes for the Council on Diabetes in Pregnancy of the American Diabetes Association. Task Force members were Richard Abrams, MD (Chair); Nancy Cooper, RD; Donald Coustan, MD; Priscilla Hollander, MD; Lois Jovanovic, MD; Daniel Lorber, MD; Boyd Metzger, MD; and Candace Wason, RN, MS.

The manuscript of the first edition was reviewed by Charles M. Clark, Jr., MD; Steven Gabbe, MD; Alan M. Golichowski, MD; Keith Johansen, MD; Ronald Kalkhoff, MD; Roger Nelson, MD; Pasquale J. Palumbo, MD; and Kathleen Wishner, PhD, MD.

We are grateful to Lois Jovanovic, MD, for reviewing this book in its second, third, fourth, and fifth editions. We thank Carol Homko, RN, CDE, MS, for reviewing the fourth edition and Laura Hieronymus, MSEd, APRN, BC-ADM, CDE, for reviewing the fifth edition. Jessica Webb, RN, BSN, CCE, and Clara Schneider, MS, RD, RN, LD, CDE, generously provided updates for this edition.

This book is dedicated to Norbert Freinkel, MD, for his superb scientific contributions to our knowledge of gestational diabetes.

Gestational diabetes is a condition that requires individualized treatment. The American Diabetes Association strongly encourages women with this condition to seek qualified medical help and to work with their health care practitioners to develop a program to manage their specific condition.

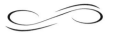

Introduction

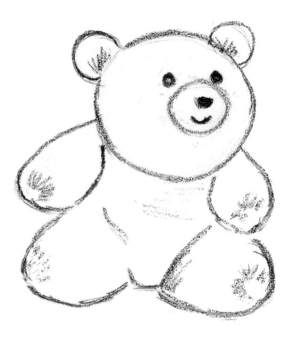

You have a lot to look forward to with the arrival of your new baby, and you shouldn't let gestational diabetes get in the way. But you can't just forget about it, either. Special care is needed during this time to keep you and your baby healthy. That's what this book is all about—helping you understand what you need to do to stay healthy and have a healthy baby.

Chapter 1

Gestational Diabetes and You

If you are like most women, you probably had never heard of gestational diabetes until you were told you had it. Gestation is another word for pregnancy, and gestational diabetes is a form of diabetes that occurs during pregnancy.

Discovering that you have gestational diabetes may have been a shock to you and your partner. You probably have many questions about it—including what gestational diabetes is, what kind of care you will need, how it will affect the health of your baby, and whether you will still have diabetes after your baby is born. In this book, we'll answer these and other questions you may have about gestational diabetes.

Besides answering your questions, this book will also help you understand what you need to do to manage gestational diabetes. Managing gestational diabetes means working to keep your blood glucose levels (the amount of sugar in your blood) within a normal range. By a normal blood glucose level, we mean the same level as a pregnant woman who does not have diabetes. Many women can control their blood glucose levels by changing their eating and exercise habits. Others may also need to take insulin.

Sometimes this change in lifestyle may seem difficult, and you will need help. Managing gestational diabetes means getting excellent medical care to be sure that the baby's special needs are met. This is where your health care team comes into play.

What is a health care team? It is a group of health professionals who are experts in different areas of your care. Before you had gestational diabetes, your team may have consisted only of your doctor. Now, because you have gestational diabetes, you may need to expand that team of health care professionals. For example, you may be asked to consult with an endocrinologist (a physician who specializes in the care of people who have diabetes). Another expert you may want to add as part of your team is a dietitian. A dietitian will help you design meal plans that will meet your body's unique nutritional needs while you have gestational diabetes. A nurse educator may also be a part of your team. This person will be able to advise you in how to manage your diabetes and will help you learn self-care techniques.

Your team can also help after your baby is born. About one-half of all women who have had gestational diabetes eventually develop diabetes, sometimes years after their babies are born. For this reason, yearly follow-up tests for diabetes are important. You should also be monitored closely if you become pregnant again, because you will be at high risk for developing gestational diabetes again. It is a good idea to continue eating nutritious foods and exercising regularly. Your team can help design programs that will fit your needs and promote optimal health after pregnancy.

Doing what you need to do to keep your blood glucose levels on target won't be easy—it will take commitment. And it will help if your partner is committed as well. Part of that commitment is understanding what you must do to achieve that goal. The fact that you're reading this book shows that you want to know more and that you care about your health and the health of your baby. We hope this book will answer most of your questions, but it isn't a substitute for your health care team. The guidelines in this book are general. Only your health care team (doctors, dietitian, and nurse educator) can suggest a program that fits your individual needs.

You—the woman with gestational diabetes—are the most important member of the health care team because you are in charge. You must keep in touch with your health care team to let them know how you are doing and whether you need help.

If you don't already have a health care team in place, your doctor may be a good source to help you find other health care providers to meet your specific needs. Your local or national American Diabetes Association office may also be able to help, and many hospitals have listings of health care professionals.

The team approach was developed with people who have diabetes in mind. It recognizes that people with diabetes are not sick but, rather, require special guidance in maintaining their health.

Do not hesitate to contact your health care providers when you have questions. Remember, they are there to help you.

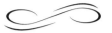

Stages of Pregnancy

Your body has already gone through numerous changes to accommodate the needs of the baby developing inside you. Each stage of your baby's development is important, and your health plays a big role in that development. The best way to take care of your baby before birth is to continue to take good care of yourself. If you are healthy, chances are your baby will be healthy, too. That's why regular checkups with members of your health care team are so important. You can take good care of your baby by taking good care of yourself.

Chapter 2

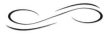

The Developing Baby

A normal pregnancy lasts 40 weeks or about 10 lunar or 9 solar months. Pregnancy—technically known as gestation—is broken down into 3 three-month periods called *trimesters*. If you were just diagnosed with gestational diabetes, you probably are at the end of the second trimester or the beginning of the third trimester. (A screening test for gestational diabetes is usually given between 24 and 28 weeks.) In all likelihood you did not have gestational diabetes during the first trimester—the time when all the major organs of the developing baby are formed and when birth defects can occur. Therefore, gestational diabetes does not put your baby at increased risk for birth defects. Instead, the risk for birth defects is probably no different than in the general population—about 2 to 3% of all births. However, some women may have had diabetes before pregnancy and not have known it. Undiagnosed type 2 diabetes before pregnancy does increase the risk of birth defects. Talk to your health care team if you think you had diabetes before becoming pregnant.

Each stage of pregnancy is exciting, as your baby slowly develops and gains all the physical characteristics he or she needs to live outside the womb. To give you an idea of your baby's progress so far and what will occur during the rest of your pregnancy, we will describe the different stages of development that normally occur during each trimester.

The First Trimester

The first five weeks of this trimester are known as the ovum or egg stage. During this stage, the fertilized egg forms the beginnings of the placenta and attaches itself to the mother's uterine wall. The placenta is the organ that links the mother's bloodstream and the baby's bloodstream. Your baby receives nourishment through the placenta.

During the first few weeks, your baby's heart forms and begins pumping blood. The digestive system, backbone, spinal cord, and brain also begin to form.

Around the eighth week, the baby will have eyes (but the lids are still joined together), a nose, lips, and a tongue. Arms, elbows, forearms, hands, knees, lower legs, and feet begin to form. Before the ninth week, your baby is technically known as an *embryo*. By the end of the embryo stage, all major organs are formed.

After the ninth week, the baby is called a *fetus*. The fetal period is devoted to growth and maturing of the organs. By the end of the first trimester, the baby will be about 3 inches long and weigh about 1 1/2 ounces. The buds and sockets for teeth in the jawbones begin to form. Fingernails and toenails start to develop, earlobes

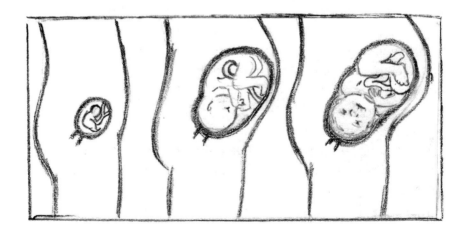

Gestational Diabetes: What to Expect

are formed, and the baby will have most of his or her organs and tissues.

The Second Trimester

The baby continues to grow and develop. About a month into the second trimester (at about 4 months), the baby will weigh about 7 ounces and will be about 6 to 7 inches long. Although the baby's heartbeat can be detected with special ultrasound equipment as early as the seventh or eighth week of pregnancy, by the fourth month it becomes strong and can be heard with either a stethoscope or a Doppler device that amplifies the sound. The baby's muscles and bones are formed. Hair grows on the head and eyebrows begin to appear. And you may start to feel the baby move at approximately 18 weeks!

Near the end of the second trimester (6 months) the baby will weigh close to 1 3/4 pounds and might be 11 to 14 inches long. The eyelids will separate and eyelashes will form. The fingernails grow to the ends of the baby's fingers. You will notice your baby's movements more.

The Third Trimester

All vital organs are fully formed. The bones in the baby's head are soft and flexible. Your baby will now begin to gain weight and grow rapidly. By the end of the seventh month, your baby will weigh 2 1/2 to 3 pounds and be 14 to 17 inches long. By the time your baby is ready to be delivered, he or she ideally will weigh about 7 to 8 1/2 pounds and be close to 20 inches long.

Chapter 3

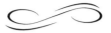

What Is Gestational Diabetes?

Gestational diabetes is a form of diabetes that appears during pregnancy (gestation) and usually disappears after pregnancy. For this reason, gestational diabetes is unlike any other type of diabetes. To help you understand gestational diabetes, let's discuss what diabetes is and the different types.

Diabetes is a disease in which the body either does not produce insulin or does not use insulin as it should. Insulin is a hormone made by the pancreas that helps deliver glucose—a form of sugar made from the food you eat—to your body's cells. Your cells use the glucose as energy, which is needed to perform all the tasks of daily living. Without insulin, glucose can't enter the cells to be used for energy. Insulin acts like a key that unlocks the door to the cells to let glucose in. When glucose cannot enter the cells, it builds up in the bloodstream, which is not healthy for you and your baby.

There are two types of diabetes that occur in people who are not pregnant: type 1 and type 2. However, when a woman with either type becomes pregnant, she needs expert medical care. Type 1 diabetes affects between 500,000 and 1 million Americans. People who have type 1 diabetes need to inject insulin daily to survive. This is because their bodies produce little or no insulin, so there is no key to unlock the door to the cells. They watch the types and amounts of food they eat. (This is known as meal planning.) In addition, they need to exercise on a regular basis. This daily routine helps them manage their diabetes. The goal of diabetes management is to keep blood glucose levels as close to normal as possible. In other words, the aim is to keep blood glucose from going too high (called hyperglycemia) or too low (called hypoglycemia).

Approximately 17 million Americans have type 2 diabetes. In type 2 diabetes, a person's body produces insulin but does not use it properly. For some reason, the body is resistant to the insulin—the key no longer fits the lock to open the door and let the glucose in. Most people are able to manage type 2 diabetes through meal planning and exercise. However, some need to take oral medication or inject insulin.

Gestational diabetes is the third type of diabetes, and it affects between 2 and 14% of all pregnant women, depending on ethnicity and other factors. The exact cause of this condition is not known. Experts do have some clues. During pregnancy, the placenta (the organ that nourishes the baby while it's growing inside the mother) produces large amounts of hormones. Hormones are important for the baby's growth. Sometimes these hormones may also block insulin's action in the mother's body, causing temporary insulin resistance that lasts until the baby is born. Today we know that all pregnant women experience some level of temporary insulin resistance, but their blood glucose stays within normal limits because the pancreas increases insulin production to compensate for this increased resistance.

Gestational diabetes develops when a woman's pancreas is unable to produce enough insulin to cover her body's needs during pregnancy. Her body cannot convert the glucose in her bloodstream into energy, so it builds up. Having too much glucose in the blood—or hyperglycemia—is how we can diagnose gestational diabetes. High blood glucose is common to type 1, type 2, and gestational diabetes. Thus all three types of diabetes require special attention to achieving and maintaining normal glucose levels.

Gestational diabetes is thought to appear around the 24th week of pregnancy, when the placenta begins producing large amounts of hormones that cause insulin resistance. Fortunately, for most

Gestational Diabetes: What to Expect

women the diabetes goes away after pregnancy because the factors that caused the insulin resistance are gone and blood glucose levels return to normal. There is a higher risk that you will have gestational diabetes in any future pregnancies, and you will need to be monitored carefully during those pregnancies. It is also very important that you have regular checkups throughout your life to detect any signs of type 2 diabetes. More than half of women with gestational diabetes will develop type 2 diabetes later in life. The way to decrease your chances of developing type 2 is to eat sensibly, achieve and maintain a healthy weight, and exercise.

How Do You Know You Have Gestational Diabetes?

Gestational diabetes is difficult to detect without a blood test because there are usually no outward signs or symptoms. Many health care providers recommend that all pregnant women be screened for gestational diabetes around 24 weeks' gestation. If you are at higher risk for developing gestational diabetes, you may be asked to take a test earlier than the 24th week. The factors placing women at higher risk for gestational diabetes and thus requiring earlier testing include the following:

- obesity
- older maternal age
- family history of diabetes
- member of an ethnic group with a high prevalence of diabetes (e.g., Latino, Native American, Asian American, African American, or Pacific Islander)
- complications in previous pregnancies, such as macrosomia (large-for-age baby), congenital malformations, and stillbirth

The first step is a test called a glucose challenge. For this test you are asked to drink a glucose solution. One hour later, your blood is tested to measure the level of glucose. If your blood glucose is below a certain standard (140 mg/dl), you do not have gestational diabetes at this time. The test may be repeated later in your pregnancy if your doctor feels there is a high risk of your developing gestational diabetes.

On the other hand, if your blood glucose level is above 140 mg/dl, you may have gestational diabetes. Your health care provider will arrange for you to have another test, called a glucose tolerance test. The glucose tolerance test is similar to the challenge test, but it takes three hours. You may eat your regular diet in the days leading up to the test. (You may be provided with specific instructions from your doctor or the laboratory.) You will be asked not to eat or drink anything but water, from after dinner the night before the test until you complete the test.

First, you will have a sample of your blood drawn. This is called a fasting blood glucose sample. After the sample is taken, you will be asked to drink a larger amount of the glucose solution than you did for the challenge test. Your blood glucose level will then be measured once every hour for three hours. Your provider will interpret the results to determine whether you have gestational diabetes. Because you can still develop gestational diabetes in the last months of pregnancy, you might be asked to repeat the tolerance test around 32 weeks' gestation.

Even if gestational diabetes is diagnosed after the 30th week, it is never too late to take steps to manage your blood glucose and improve the outcome of your pregnancy. As you age, your chances of developing gestational diabetes increase. Therefore, just because you didn't have gestational diabetes during your first pregnancy doesn't mean you won't develop it in later pregnancies.

Potential Problems for the Baby

Although your baby is not at greater risk for birth defects, gestational diabetes can still create some problems for your baby. Most of these problems can be prevented by taking precautions to keep you and your baby healthy. Let's discuss some of the problems common among babies born to women with gestational diabetes whose blood glucose levels are higher than normal.

Macrosomia

Macrosomia literally means "large body" and refers to a baby who is larger than normal for its developmental age. Women with gestational diabetes whose blood glucose levels are higher than normal are more likely to have macrosomic babies. This occurs because the babies receive nourishment by absorbing glucose and other nutrients from the mother's blood through the placenta. If your blood glucose levels are high, your nutrient levels will be much higher than normal, and the baby will receive more glucose than he or she needs.

When "fed" the extra glucose, a baby tends to get fat. Because the baby does not have diabetes, its pancreas will produce extra insulin to use all the blood glucose. The extra insulin the baby is forced to produce makes it grow bigger and fatter.

Delivery of a large baby can be difficult for both the mother and the child. During a vaginal birth of a large baby, there is a chance that the baby's shoulders will be injured or that the baby will be deprived of oxygen for a period of time. Sometimes a baby may be too large to be delivered vaginally, and a cesarean delivery will be necessary. There are tests, such as ultrasounds, that might help your provider estimate the size of your baby and determine the safest method of delivery. In addition to the difficulties during pregnancy and delivery, babies with macrosomia face an increased risk for future obesity and type 2 diabetes.

Hypoglycemia (Low Blood Glucose)

If your blood glucose level is too high right before or during labor, your baby's pancreas will make extra insulin to balance the extra glucose he or she is getting from you. After delivery, however, when your baby is no longer getting its glucose from you, the extra insulin it produced can cause the baby's own blood glucose level to fall below normal limits. If the low blood glucose is not treated, it can cause serious problems for the newborn. If necessary, the baby can be given glucose in a bottle or through an intravenous line (IV) and watched carefully in the hospital nursery.

Jaundice

Jaundice is a yellowing of the skin caused by a waste product called bilirubin. Before birth, your baby needs a large supply of red blood cells. At birth, your baby no longer needs this extra supply, so its liver breaks down and excretes the old red blood cells.

Your baby's liver may have trouble handling this workload. This can cause a buildup of red blood cells. The broken-down red blood cells are called bilirubin. Instead of being excreted, bilirubin is deposited in the baby's tissues, causing a condition called jaundice. It's the bilirubin that colors the skin yellow.

It is common for babies to be born with small amounts of bilirubin in their system. If they build up large amounts of bilirubin soon after birth they may need to be fed formula with a bottle or be exposed to special lights. Digesting food and exposure to the lights can help break down and get rid of bilirubin. In most children who develop jaundice, this treatment is successful and lasts only a few days. High levels of bilirubin can be harmful, but thankfully, such occurrences are rare.

If jaundice becomes severe, the baby might need a blood transfusion. Since jaundice is more common in babies whose mothers have diabetes, your health care team will pay special attention to the possibility of jaundice in your newborn.

Respiratory Distress Syndrome (RDS)

Because babies of mothers with diabetes tend to gain more weight than is normal (see "Macrosomia," page 17), these babies have an increased risk of being born prematurely (before 37 weeks' gestation). With prematurity and other possible diabetes-related factors, these babies are at risk for respiratory distress syndrome (RDS). In babies with RDS, the lungs have not developed enough for the baby to breathe on its own. A baby born with RDS is cared for in the intensive care unit until the baby can breathe on its own. Newborns with RDS are given oxygen and surfactant (a substance that expands the lungs) to help them breathe. Before delivery, your doctor may recommend a test called amniocentesis (see page 58), which will tell the doctor the degree of maturity of the baby's lungs and indicate the baby's risk for developing RDS. Your provider may also suggest that you get an injection of betamethasone, a steroid, before delivery to help increase the baby's lung maturity.

Potential Problems for the Mother

Your health care provider will explain and help you set up a program to keep your blood glucose level within a normal range. This program will be designed especially for you and may include meal planning, exercise, and possibly insulin therapy. Following this program will help you keep your blood glucose level on track and help you stay healthy. Women with gestational diabetes may face an increased risk for three problems—preeclampsia, urinary tract infections, and ketonuria.

Preeclampsia

Preeclampsia is the technical name for pregnancy-induced high blood pressure, which is frequently accompanied by swelling, often in the hands and face, headache, blurred vision, and pain in the upper stomach (like heartburn). High blood pressure is not good for you or your baby and can be life threatening. Your health care team will work with you to treat this condition. Treatments vary from limiting activity to hospitalization. This condition usually goes away shortly after your baby is born.

Urinary Tract Infections

Urinary tract infections can be more common among women with gestational diabetes. Symptoms include burning on urination, frequency of urination, and urgency (needing to go immediately). These infections are treated with antibiotics prescribed by your health care team. Be sure to drink 6 to 8 glasses of water each day. Coffee, tea, and sodas don't count because they remove water from your system. Be sure to discuss this potential health problem, its treatments, and ways to prevent it with your health care team.

Ketonuria

Ketones are acid substances that are produced when your body breaks down fat because no other source of energy is available. Excess ketones build up in the blood and are excreted in the urine, a condition called ketonuria. During pregnancy, this usually means you are not eating enough for both you and your baby. Ketones are monitored because they can cross the placenta and enter your baby's blood. Large amounts of ketones are harmful to your baby. At your office visits, your urine will be checked for ketones, and your provider may also suggest that you check your urine at home in the mornings. You will urinate into a specimen cup and use a test strip dipped into the urine to check for the presence of ketones. If your provider asks you to do this, you will be given specific instructions on when and how often to check your urine. You can buy ketone test strips at a pharmacy.

In general, to prevent ketones from developing, it is important to keep your blood glucose levels on target by following your meal plan, exercising, and taking insulin if necessary. If you have any ketones in your urine and your blood glucose levels are normal, you may need to eat extra calories each day. Ask your doctor or diabetes educator what to do if you have ketones in your urine.

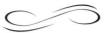

Treatment

Discovering that you have gestational diabetes may have been a shock to you and your partner. It is enough just to worry about having a baby without having to worry about a condition you know little about. But you shouldn't worry—gestational diabetes is manageable. That's good news because it means that, with some planning and effort, you and your baby can be as healthy as ever.

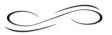

Chapter 4

Nutrition

Good nutritional habits play an important role in any pregnancy. But when you have gestational diabetes, the amount and types of food you eat play an even more important role. The food you eat raises your blood glucose level. If you eat more than is recommended, your blood glucose level may become too high. High blood glucose levels are not healthy for you or your baby.

For many women, eating a well-balanced diet is enough to keep their blood glucose levels within a normal range and provide the needed nutrients for their babies. Some exercise will also be a part of your treatment program. Other women with gestational diabetes will need to inject insulin every day until their baby is born to keep glucose levels close to normal. In this case, you need to match the food you eat with the amount and timing of the insulin you inject and the exercise you do. If you are injecting insulin, it is important to know what you eat, when you eat, and how much you eat. Regardless of how you manage your gestational diabetes, following a meal plan is important.

A meal plan will help you eat the right amounts and types of foods. A dietitian or your health care team can help you design a meal plan especially for you. Your meal plan should include foods you prefer that also meet your diabetes and pregnancy needs. See the appendix for more information about meal planning and sample meals. If you don't already have a dietitian and don't know where to look for one, your doctor, your hospital, or the American Diabetes Association (ADA) may have a listing of registered dietitians (RD) in your area. (Call 1-800-DIABETES for help from the ADA in finding an RD.)

Everyone can benefit from healthy meal planning—but this is especially true for mothers-to-be. And since it is so important, let's discuss what you need to do to meet your nutritional needs and those of your baby throughout the rest of your pregnancy.

Meal Planning for a Healthy Baby

Your nutritional needs change during pregnancy for two reasons. First, your baby needs nourishment. Second, your body will change the way it uses certain nutrients. If you haven't been doing so already, you should start practicing good nutrition to fulfill the needs of your baby before birth as well as during lactation (breast-feeding). To help you understand the importance of good nutrition, let's look at the nutritional needs of your baby while he or she is developing and growing inside you.

Your Baby's Needs

The growth and development of a baby has a lot to do with the mother's nutritional habits and weight gain. Although losing weight while you're pregnant is not recommended, following a well-balanced meal plan is. Here's why: When the mother doesn't get all the nutrients she needs—either because food is scarce or because she chooses not to eat enough—her supply of nutrients to her baby is reduced. The mother's body tries to protect itself from "starvation" before it protects the baby.

This is particularly true in the second half of pregnancy. The consequences of the mother's poor nutrition may include health problems for the baby. Poor nutrition can also affect the placenta, which performs several tasks that are essential to the baby's health. The placenta transports many substances—including glucose, amino acids, and hormones—from the mother's system to the baby's system. If you are poorly nourished, the placenta cannot perform these functions properly. Part of meeting your nutritional needs is making sure you gain enough weight.

Weight Gain during Pregnancy

A weight gain of 25 to 32 pounds is considered appropriate for mothers who are at a normal weight when they become pregnant. If you were overweight before pregnancy, your health care team may have recommended that you gain less than 15 pounds. If you were underweight before pregnancy, you may have been encouraged to gain slightly more weight.

Just how much weight you need to gain is something your health care team may have already determined, based on your body and your baby's needs. It is important to remember that pregnancy is not a time to lose weight. A meal plan that is too low in calories may deprive your baby of the nutrients it needs to develop and grow properly.

For an average-sized woman, weight gain is quite small during the first three months—only about 2 to 4 pounds. A woman who is underweight needs to gain more than this, in part to build up adequate fat stores. Fat stores act as a reserve to provide for the added energy needs of you and your baby. In addition, fat stores aid in providing nutrition during lactation. About 7 to 10 pounds of weight gain during pregnancy come from an increase in fat stores. If you are overweight, less fat stores will be needed.

If you are past the second trimester, you may have noticed that you are gaining weight at a much faster rate—about a pound a week on average. This pattern of weight gain tends to result in the best outcome of pregnancy.

Rather than focusing on the total weight you gain, it is more important to consider your pattern of weight gain. If you start to gain a lot of weight suddenly or if you stop gaining weight or even start losing weight, your health care team will want to know why.

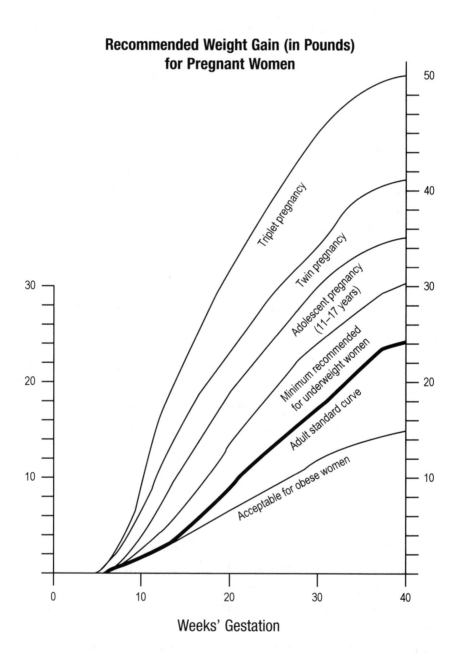

Recommended Weight Gain (in Pounds) for Pregnant Women

Triplet pregnancy

Twin pregnancy

Adolescent pregnancy (11–17 years)

Minimum recommended for underweight women

Adult standard curve

Acceptable for obese women

Weeks' Gestation

Gestational Diabetes: What to Expect

At your prenatal appointments your weight will be checked and your health care team and you will discuss any abnormal weight changes. The problem could be caused by excess fluid retention or may be related to the food you eat and may be easily solved by making changes in what you eat.

Weight Gain for Overweight Mothers

Mothers who are overweight during pregnancy might have problems. By overweight we mean women who are more than 20% over their ideal body weight before becoming pregnant. The problems overweight women may face can include an increased incidence of hypertension (high blood pressure) and preeclampsia (hypertension and swelling caused by pregnancy). If you are obese, weight gain during pregnancy should probably be less than 15 pounds.

If you had weight problems before pregnancy, now is not the time to lose weight. The time to lose weight is later—after delivery. If you don't eat enough calories now, your system may be forced to burn more fat than usual. This will produce ketones (called starvation ketosis), and ketones could be harmful to your baby. So weight loss during pregnancy should be avoided.

Weight Gain for Underweight Mothers

About 10% of all women who become pregnant are underweight at the time of pregnancy. Another 10% become underweight because they do not eat properly during pregnancy. It is important to gain the proper weight to reduce the risk of having a baby with a low birth weight. However, there is no proof that forcing yourself to gain weight will also cause your baby to gain weight. So how much should you gain? The answer is whatever your body needs to ensure a safe pregnancy. Check with your health care team for advice.

Adolescents and Pregnancy

Teenagers who become pregnant may need to eat more calories than most other women. Because the body of a teenager is still growing, the teen mother needs to provide for her body's own needs for growth as well as for her baby's. Your health care practitioner can help you determine a weight goal.

Distribution of Weight Gain

During the early part of your pregnancy, your baby will gain very little weight—not much more than 1 gram (about 1/28 of an ounce) of body weight per day. You will also gain little weight during this time, but your body will start to change dramatically. Your breasts and uterus enlarge, your blood volume expands, and the placenta and amniotic fluid form.

The fat stores in your body will also increase rapidly. One of the first things you may notice when you become pregnant is a gradual thickening of your waist, back, and upper thighs. This process is both natural and important. It occurs because your body is storing nutrients so that there are some reserves available to safeguard the nutritional needs of your baby in the following months.

For the first four months, your baby's daily nutrient needs are very small. However, by the sixth month, your baby will gain about 10 times more weight each day than it gained early in pregnancy.

Nutrient Needs

Pregnant women have specific nutrient needs. Your diet should include complex carbohydrates, especially those high in fiber, such as beans and starchy vegetables, whole-grain breads, and fruits. You should also cut down on the fat in your diet. The following are some of the nutrients you will need during your pregnancy.

Carbohydrates

Although there are no specific guidelines for the amount of daily carbohydrates a woman with gestational diabetes should eat, most women do well when about 40 to 45% of daily calories come from carbohydrates. The best way to ensure that you are eating the right amount, however, is to test your glucose levels. Your fasting blood glucose should register 90 mg/dl or less, and one hour after a meal your blood glucose should measure 120 mg/dl or less. (The abbreviation "mg/dl" means milligrams of glucose per deciliter of blood. It is a standard way of measuring blood glucose levels.)

When you have gestational diabetes, the type of carbohydrate you eat is just as important as the amount you eat. The recommended carbohydrates are starches, or complex carbohydrates, such as vegetables, beans, pasta, whole grains, tortillas, rice, and wheat breads. Concentrated sweets, such as table sugar, cookies, candy, sodas, Jell-o, fruit juice, and pastries are both high in calories and low in nutrients. They can contribute to obesity in the mother-to-be and to macrosomia in her baby, so they should be avoided.

Some women with gestational diabetes who take insulin may find that eating the same amount of carbohydrates at the same meals can help them manage their blood glucose. It's the carbohydrate in your meals that raises your blood glucose.

Fiber

Most fiber is an indigestible form of carbohydrate that is highly recommended for pregnant women. Fiber delays the absorption of nutrients from the intestine and allows the blood glucose to rise gradually after a meal. Fiber also reduces constipation that often occurs during pregnancy.

Protein

About 20 to 25% of your daily calories should come from protein. Good sources for protein are milk and other dairy products, meat, poultry, fish, and legumes (dried beans and peas). During pregnancy, protein helps expand your blood volume and promotes growth of breast and uterine tissues. It is especially important for the growth and development of your baby.

Fat

About 30 to 40% of your daily calories should come from fat. Unfortunately, most people eat too much fat. Fats are high in calories, so they need to be limited. Fat is found in meats, dairy products, snack foods, butter, margarine, peanut butter, salad dressings, oils, and nuts. Be sure to ask your dietitian for tips on how to limit your fat intake to equal 40% of your daily calories. The healthiest fats are canola or olive oil and small amounts of butter. The hydrogenated fats in margarine and snack foods are not good for you.

Vitamins

Eating a well-balanced diet will usually provide the vitamins and minerals you need while you are pregnant. However, you may not get the amount of iron, calcium, and folic acid you and your baby need. For this reason, your health care practitioner may ask you to take prenatal vitamin supplements.

There are two reasons why you need more iron while you are pregnant: to provide for your increase in blood production and to supply iron to your baby, so he or she can produce blood.

Babies store the iron they receive in their livers. If your diet is rich in iron, your baby will be born with enough iron stores to last through the months when he or she is fed mainly milk. (Milk, unless fortified, does not contain iron.) Most foods don't contain enough iron for you to get the amount you need during pregnancy. So unless you are willing to eat liver once or twice a week, your health care provider will most likely ask you to take an iron supplement.

You also need to get enough calcium during pregnancy. The recommended intake is 1,000 mg per day (1,300 mg for women under age 19). Calcium is important for bone development and strength. Milk is an excellent source of calcium. One quart of milk or the equivalent in other milk products (such as four cartons of yogurt) will give you the calcium you need. If you are not able to drink that much milk or if you are allergic to milk, you may need to take a calcium supplement, preferably calcium carbonate. Ask your doctor or dietitian about calcium supplements.

You can get a sufficient amount of calcium by drinking vitamin D–fortified milk and through exposure of skin to sunlight. Vitamin D is important along with calcium because it promotes calcium absorption.

Another important vitamin to take prior to conception and during pregnancy is folic acid, which has been shown to prevent certain birth defects. It is common in a variety of foods, but you will likely need to take supplements since you will need almost twice the usual requirement while you're pregnant. Some good sources of folic acid include dark green leafy vegetables (spinach or kale), dried beans, liver, oranges, and whole-wheat products.

The need for other vitamins (such as the B vitamins or vitamin C) increases only slightly during pregnancy. Too much of some vitamins, such as vitamin A, can be harmful to both you and your baby. Ask your health care practitioner for specific guidelines.

Dietary Precautions

There are some dietary precautions recommended by the U.S. Food and Drug Administration for all pregnant women.

Mercury. You should avoid fish and shellfish that contain high levels of mercury. Do not eat shark, swordfish, king mackerel, or tilefish while you are pregnant. Limit the amount of white tuna or albacore you eat to 6 ounces a week. You can eat up to 12 ounces a week of low-mercury fish, such as flounder, haddock, herring, sardines, scallop, shrimp, and tilapia.

PCBs. Polychlorinated biphenyls (PCBs) are a type of highly toxic industrial compound found in some seafood. Fatty fish such as salmon, bluefish, striped bass, pike, trout, and walleye may contain PCBs. Check with your supermarket and state fish and wildlife agencies to find your regional precautions.

Bacteria. Some foods are more likely to harbor harmful bacteria. Do not eat raw or undercooked meat, seafood, or eggs. Avoid soft cheeses like blue cheese, feta, brie, Roquefort, blue-veined, queso blanco, queso fresco, panela, and Camembert, unless the label indicates that the cheese has been pasteurized. Hard cheeses, processed cheeses, and cream and cottage cheese are fine.

The March of Dimes recommends reheating deli meat, hot dogs, and packaged luncheon meats to 165 degrees Fahrenheit to kill harmful bacteria. You may eat canned pâtés and canned smoked seafood but not the refrigerated varieties. Avoid any unpasteurized milk or juice products, as well as raw vegetable sprouts.

Food preparation. Pregnant women need to make sure that their food has been handled safely. Food handlers should carefully wash their hands, as well as cooking tools and work surfaces. Wash fruits and vegetables well before eating. Throw away the outer leaves of lettuce and cabbage. Never eat cooked food that has been left unrefrigerated for more than 2 hours.

Putting It All Together

You probably still have questions—about artificial sweeteners, alcohol, caffeine, and other substances, as well as about when to eat and how much. Some of that information is addressed below, but you should talk with your dietitian or other members of your health care team for guidelines that are specific for you.

Eat small, frequent meals. Eating smaller meals more often during the day can help prevent high blood glucose after meals. Experts recommend three small meals and three snacks a day to keep you from becoming overly hungry. Frequent meals can also help you avoid the nausea and heartburn that many pregnant women experience. If you include a protein food with every meal and snack, you'll get double benefits: Protein is digested and absorbed more slowly than carbohydrates are, so you will feel satisfied longer and you'll run less risk of hyperglycemia (high blood glucose).

Eat a small breakfast. Morning blood glucose levels are likely to be high if you have gestational diabetes, so it is best to avoid fruits and juices and eat a small breakfast of whole grains and protein-rich foods.

Saccharin and aspartame. Some women may be concerned about whether it is safe to use artificial sweeteners, such as saccharin and aspartame (Equal or NutraSweet), during pregnancy. Because saccharin can cross the placenta to the baby, it may be a risk for pregnant women. Saccharin should be avoided during pregnancy.

Aspartame is composed of the amino acids aspartate and phenylalanine. Aspartame seems to cause little concern for pregnant women, because these two amino acids are found in most of the protein we eat. It is unlikely that eating or drinking an average amount (such as one can of diet soda or one serving of aspartame-sweetened dessert per day) would be harmful.

Sucralose. Sucralose (Splenda) is a noncaloric sweetener made from sugar. Current research has allowed use in all populations, including pregnant women and nursing mothers. Sucralose may be beneficial for individuals with diabetes because research demonstrates that sucralose has no effect on carbohydrate metabolism, short- or long-term blood glucose control, or insulin secretion. There are a variety of Splenda products available in the supermarket, including carbonated soft drinks, low-calorie fruit drinks, maple syrup, and applesauce. This may be a good sugar substitute for you during pregnancy and can be reviewed with your health care team.

Caffeine. Caffeine is a colorless, bitter substance that works as a stimulant, which means that it increases the activity of the heart and central nervous system. It is found in coffee and tea and in many carbonated beverages. In 1981, the U.S. Food and Drug Administration issued a general warning encouraging women to avoid unnecessary caffeine consumption during pregnancy, although an NIH-NICHD study showed that moderate caffeine consumption is safe. It's probably a good idea for pregnant women who choose to use caffeine to do so in moderation. (Moderation for you may not be the same as moderation for another woman. Ask your health care provider how much caffeine is safe for you.)

Alcohol. Today, we know that it can be dangerous to drink alcohol during pregnancy. Women who drink alcohol regularly during pregnancy have a greater risk of delivering a baby with birth defects. Some examples of birth defects are unusual facial characteristics, low birth weight, and defects in the baby's central nervous system that could result in a decrease in intellectual abilities, perhaps even mental retardation.

It appears that low doses of alcohol—such as two glasses of beer a night—if consumed regularly by the mother, may result in growth failure and/or lower IQ in her baby. Even moderate amounts of alcohol seem to double the risk of a miscarriage, as well as growth failure of the baby. No one knows if there is a safe level of alcohol consumption during pregnancy.

The best advice for all pregnant women is to drink no alcohol.

Smoking. Besides being unhealthy for you, cigarette smoking can also be harmful to your baby. Smoking can contribute to your baby having a low birth weight. In contrast to alcohol, most of the growth retardation due to smoking occurs during the last three months of pregnancy. Stopping smoking even as late as the last few months may reduce its harmful effect. Smoking will not affect your weight gain, but it can affect your baby's.

The more a mother smokes, the higher her risk for problems. If you can't stop smoking, you should at least try to cut back on the number of cigarettes you smoke. The earlier a mother stops smoking and the less she smokes the better.

Cocaine and other drugs. While you are pregnant, it is very important that you use only the medications specifically prescribed for you. While so-called "recreational drugs," such as cocaine, are harmful for you at any time, use of these drugs during pregnancy can result in harmful effects for your baby. Some of the problems that can result from using these drugs include birth of an underweight and undersized baby, mental retardation, and abruption of the placenta (premature separation of the placenta from the uterus, a life-threatening condition for the baby). We advise that you totally avoid any harmful drugs during pregnancy.

How to Handle Problems That Accompany Pregnancy

While you are pregnant, you may not always feel as well as you'd like. Here are a few ideas on how to handle some of the common problems that occur during pregnancy.

Nausea and vomiting. Try some of the following tips:
- Eat crackers, pretzels, or dry toast when you wake up and before you get out of bed.
- Sip small amounts (less than 8 ounces) of carbonated beverages.
- Eat smaller meals and eat more often.
- Drink fluids between meals instead of with meals.
- Avoid spicy and greasy foods.
- Avoid lying down for 30 minutes after eating.

Constipation. Constipation is common during pregnancy. One reason is that your intestinal muscles become more relaxed. Another reason is that, as your baby grows, there is more pressure on your intestines. If you have problems with constipation, try the following:

- Drink plenty of liquids, especially water.
- Eat high-fiber foods, including whole-grain breads, bran cereal, and vegetables.
- Get regular exercise. But don't overdo in a single outing.
- If the problem persists, discuss it with your doctor or health care practitioner.

Heartburn. As your pregnancy progresses, you may get heartburn. Some of the symptoms of heartburn include burning discomfort in the stomach or throat, an upset stomach, or a stomachache. The following may help:

- Eat frequent, small meals that include protein.
- Eat more foods with calcium and magnesium in them.
- Avoid acidic or spicy foods.
- Eat slowly; be sure to chew food well.
- If heartburn persists, check with your doctor or health care provider for help.

Chapter 5

Exercise and Pregnancy

In general, physical activity is good for you. It can also be harmful if you overdo it or participate in an activity that is too stressful for your body. You should listen to your body while exercising.

If you feel fatigued while working out, stop and rest. Fatigue in pregnancy is the body's way of forcing a woman to slow down and rest. It is important to discuss any exercise program with your doctor or health care practitioner before you start. This is true any time, but especially while you are pregnant. You may have already discussed an exercise program with your doctor and may have been following an exercise program since you became pregnant. If you haven't, talk with your doctor about the effects exercise can have on your pregnancy.

Even if you were physically fit before becoming pregnant, you need to be sure that your body can handle an exercise program as it adjusts to the stress of pregnancy. You may be advised to exercise at a more moderate level and to avoid certain activities until after you deliver your baby. As a general rule, your pulse should not go above 140 beats per minute, and you should not allow it to stay elevated for longer than 20 minutes per exercise session. Check with your health care provider for specific guidelines for you.

Activities you may be advised to avoid include racquet sports, volleyball, and basketball. These activities involve twists, turns, jumping, and sudden starts and stops—all of which can strain

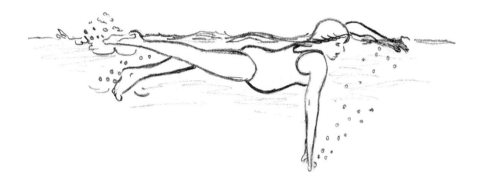

your muscles, joints, and ligaments. You should also avoid hazardous activities such as water skiing and snow skiing (you might fall at a high speed). Many women should also avoid jogging while pregnant (you might fall, and the pounding could prove harmful to your pregnancy).

While you may have to eliminate some activities during your pregnancy, there are other exercises you can do to stay fit. For example, brisk walking may be a good alternative. Many women who find jogging too strenuous have benefited from walking. A brisk walk following a meal (about 30 minutes after eating) may be ideal for keeping your blood glucose on target. This may be especially true after breakfast, since blood glucose levels are often highest in the morning.

Swimming can also be a good exercise for many pregnant women. The buoyancy of the water eases stress on the joints. Swimming isn't bone jarring or hard on your feet and legs, so you are less likely to get injured. Some areas also offer water aerobics classes.

Many areas and facilities are striving to provide prenatal exercise classes. These classes move at a slower pace and are designed with pregnant women in mind. They include classes in yoga, pilates, step, and prenatal aerobics. If you are interested and have been advised by your health care team that it is safe for you to exercise, you might find a new exercise program that you can also continue after your pregnancy.

Gestational Diabetes and Exercise

When you have gestational diabetes, your goal is to keep your blood glucose levels as close to normal as possible. In most cases, exercise lowers blood glucose by helping body cells become more sensitive to insulin, thereby overcoming insulin resistance. Because of this, exercise can be particularly helpful in keeping blood glucose levels within a normal range. To help manage gestational diabetes, you may be asked to exercise on a regular basis. For example, your health care provider may advise that you walk for 20 to 30 minutes every day after breakfast.

If You Take Insulin . . .

It is important to remember that exercise and insulin both lower blood glucose. If insulin is prescribed for you, be sure to read the sections on hypoglycemia and exercise (pages 46–48).

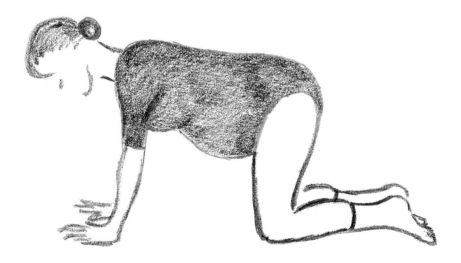

Postnatal Exercises

Remember, the need for fitness never stops—not even during the excitement of caring for your baby and rescheduling your life to meet your baby's needs. Physical activity will help your body make the major adjustments needed after pregnancy. Toning your muscles helps your body get back to the firm shape it was before you were pregnant. If you don't exercise, you may find it much harder to tighten up your body later.

You can probably start exercising soon after your baby is born, but you'll want to check with your doctor before you begin. If you have a cesarean delivery, you may have to wait a little longer. Again, ask your doctor when you can safely return to your prepregnancy exercise program or begin a new workout routine.

Chapter 6

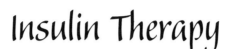

Insulin Therapy

Sometimes following a meal plan and exercising aren't enough to keep your blood glucose level within a normal range. If you are following a meal and exercise plan but your blood glucose levels remain consistently high, you may need insulin. This happens to approximately 20% of women who develop gestational diabetes. Insulin is effective only when it is injected through the skin with a syringe or insulin pen.

If insulin is the chosen treatment method for your condition, you will need to inject the insulin. It is normal to feel apprehensive about giving yourself a shot. However, with proper technique and today's very fine needles, an injection can be almost painless (see pages 43–46). This chapter will help answer some of your questions about insulin and its use.

Insulin's Role

In Chapter 3, we explained that insulin helps glucose enter your body's cells to be converted into energy. Without insulin, glucose cannot enter the cells and instead builds up in the blood, which is not healthy. Under normal conditions, a woman's pancreas produces enough insulin to meet her body's needs. But pregnancy demands more insulin than normal because of the increased production of hormones that lead to insulin resistance. With gestational diabetes, a woman's pancreas cannot produce enough insulin to overcome her body's resistance. For some women, carefully watching their food intake (following a meal plan) is enough to overcome this resistance. Some need to add exercise to the program. And still others need to inject insulin. Just what your diabetes plan entails will depend on your body's special needs. If you do need to inject insulin, it will help you to know about the different types of insulin, how they work, and how to make injections easier.

Types of Insulin

For many years, purified animal insulins were widely used by people with diabetes. Today, human insulin is used. Human insulin is identical to that produced by a human pancreas, but it is made in the laboratory. The newer insulins work quickly and are safe for use by women with gestational diabetes.

Insulins vary in their action times—the length of time they work at lowering blood glucose. There are four types of insulin that may be prescribed for women with gestational diabetes: rapid acting; regular, also called short acting; NPH, also called intermediate acting; and long acting. Your health care team will determine the type of insulin, or combination of types, that you need, and they will help you learn to monitor its effects.

Rapid-acting insulins begin acting in 10 to 30 minutes after injection. They reach their peak activity in 90 minutes and last for 3 to 5 hours. These insulins are injected right before eating and take effect very rapidly, and they are excellent for keeping after-meal blood glucose levels on target.

Regular insulins usually reach the bloodstream within 30 to 60 minutes. This type of insulin is most effective—or peaks—2 to 5 hours after you inject it. It stays in your bloodstream from 5 to 8 hours, although not at full strength.

Intermediate-acting (NPH) insulins take 1 to 2 hours to reach the bloodstream. They are the strongest 2 to 12 hours after injection and can stay in the blood up to 24 hours. Long-acting insulins take 30 minutes to 3 hours to have an initial effect and then reach their peak at 4 to 20 hours. They can remain in your system for 24 hours.

The number of daily injections you will need depends on how effective they are in lowering your blood glucose levels. Your insulin dose may change as your pregnancy progresses. For example, as you get farther along in pregnancy, your resistance to insulin tends to increase, and you may need to increase your insulin dose. Changes in your insulin dosage may be necessary as often as every 7 to 14 days.

Storing Your Insulin

Manufacturers recommend storing unopened bottles of insulin in the refrigerator. Since injecting cold insulin can sometimes make an injection more painful, you can keep the insulin you are using at room temperature (around 70ºF).

Store the extra bottles in the refrigerator. Insulin should not be exposed to extreme temperatures, so you should never store it in the freezer or in direct sunlight. When you use up the insulin in one bottle, take another from the refrigerator, so that it can be ready for your next injection. Write the date on the label, so you know how long it's been open.

Always check the expiration dates on all bottles and never use insulin with an expired date. Check the bottles of insulin to see if there are any crystals (frosting) on the bottle or in the insulin. (Keep in mind, though, that intermediate-acting insulins are usually cloudy.) If you find any of these problems, take the bottle back to the pharmacy.

Giving Yourself Injections

It is normal to be apprehensive about giving yourself a shot. But once you actually do it, you'll realize how relatively painless it can be, especially if you know some of the tricks to make an injection easier. Here's how to give yourself an injection:

1. Fill the syringe with the correct amount of insulin, and then remove the needle from the bottle carefully to make sure that no insulin is lost.
2. Wipe the area you intend to inject with alcohol and a cotton swab and let the alcohol dry completely. (This step is optional.)
3. With one hand, pinch up the skin where you are going to inject the insulin. Pinching up the skin helps you avoid injecting into a muscle, which can be painful and can affect how the insulin is absorbed. If you are injecting in the arm, you can press your arm against a chair or a wall to push up the skin, or have someone help you.
4. With your other hand, hold the syringe like you would a pencil. Insert the needle at a 90-degree angle to the injection site, using a gentle darting motion.
5. Steadily press the plunger in—do not stop and start. If you can't easily push the plunger in, pull back on the needle slightly and try again. If it won't move easily, pull the needle out and try another injection site. If the plunger still won't move, fill a new syringe. The insulin may be jamming the needle, especially if the syringe has been used repeatedly. If your injection is especially painful, you may have blunted the needle during preparation or inserted it into your skin too slowly.
6. Pull the needle straight out. Cover the injection site with your finger or a cotton ball and apply slight pressure (but do not rub) for 5 to 8 seconds.
7. Dispose of your needles in a puncture-proof, heavy-duty plastic or metal container with a lid that can be sealed shut before it is placed in the garbage. Removing the needles from the syringes when you are finished with them will prevent anyone from reusing them.

Gestational Diabetes: What to Expect

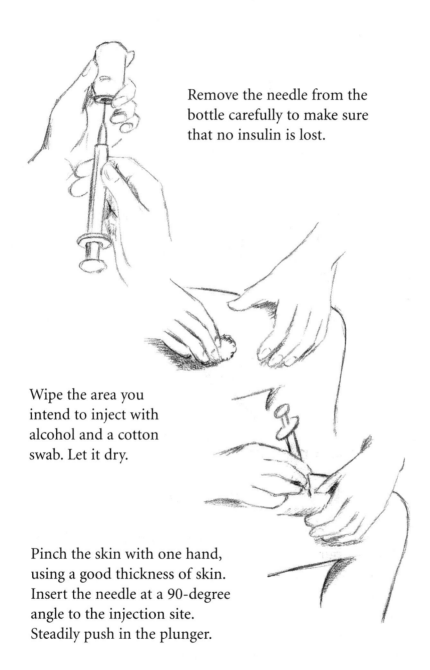

Remove the needle from the bottle carefully to make sure that no insulin is lost.

Wipe the area you intend to inject with alcohol and a cotton swab. Let it dry.

Pinch the skin with one hand, using a good thickness of skin. Insert the needle at a 90-degree angle to the injection site. Steadily push in the plunger.

Remember that a member of your health care team will be able to instruct you and answer any questions you have about giving yourself injections.

Keeping a Balance

Once insulin has been injected, it will work according to its action schedule—regardless of whether you follow yours! In other words, the insulin you inject before a meal will start lowering your blood glucose level as scheduled even if you don't eat. So, as we mentioned in Chapter 4, you need to balance the carbohydrate you eat with the insulin you inject. Exercise also plays a role in this balance. Physical activity lowers blood glucose. If you don't plan for it, exercise can lower your blood glucose level too far, causing hypoglycemia (low blood glucose).

Balancing the food you eat with your insulin dosage and the exercise you do is the key to keeping your blood glucose level as close to normal as possible. A normal fasting (or early morning) or premeal blood glucose level is under 90 mg/dl. About one hour after meals, an average blood glucose level is below 120 mg/dl, and by two hours, it is below 110 mg/dl. (These are called one-hour postprandial and two-hour postprandial readings.) These levels are considered "normal," and they are the blood glucose goals for pregnant women with gestational diabetes.

Hypoglycemia

One of the main problems for people who take insulin is hypoglycemia or low blood glucose. An episode of hypoglycemia or low blood glucose is also sometimes called an insulin reaction. Most women with gestational diabetes who take insulin will not experience hypoglycemia. Still, it helps to be aware of the causes, symptoms, and treatments, just in case.

Hypoglycemia can be caused by a number of things. Usually it happens because there is not a balance between the food you eat, the exercise you do, and the insulin you inject. Each affects blood glucose differently: insulin and exercise lower blood glucose and food raises it. If you take too large a dose of insulin, eat too little carbohydrate or don't eat on time, or unexpectedly exercise too much, your blood glucose may drop too low.

Checking your blood is the best way to know whether your blood glucose is low (see "Blood Glucose Monitoring," pages 49–51). But there are symptoms that will help you recognize an insulin reaction. The symptoms include

- shakiness or dizziness
- sweating
- clumsy or jerky movements
- hunger
- headache
- sudden moodiness or behavior changes, such as crying for no apparent reason
- pale skin color
- difficulty paying attention or confusion
- tingling sensations around the mouth

If you notice any of these symptoms, check your blood glucose. If it is low (below 70 mg/dl), eat or drink some carbohydrate. If you cannot test your blood, treat the reaction and then call your health care practitioner. It is better to have too much glucose than to have an insulin reaction.

The best treatment for hypoglycemia is 4 ounces of fruit juice or 8 ounces of milk. Other examples are 3 or 4 pieces of hard candy or sugar cubes, 2 tablespoons of raisins, or 3 or 4 glucose tablets (available at your pharmacy). Note that these are only suggestions. You should check with your dietitian or other health care practitioner for specific ways to treat a reaction. Get into the habit of carrying some form of carbohydrate with you for times when your blood glucose level is low, especially when you exercise if you are also taking insulin.

When You Exercise . . .

Because exercise and insulin both lower blood glucose, you may need to modify your exercise program if insulin is prescribed for you. To help you avoid hypoglycemia, your health care provider will want to know when and how much you exercise. Changes can include rescheduling exercise periods or meals or adding extra snacks.

When you exercise while on insulin therapy, you must take some precautions:

- Check with your health care team before you begin any exercise program when you are pregnant.
- Test your blood glucose level before and after exercising. Again, ask your health care team for specific guidelines on safe blood glucose levels before, during, and after exercise.

Chapter 7

Monitoring Gestational Diabetes

In addition to meal planning, exercising, and possibly injecting insulin, you will be asked to check your blood glucose. Knowing your blood glucose level will help you know how well you are managing your gestational diabetes. The results of the tests will help you and your health care team make adjustments to keep you and your baby healthy.

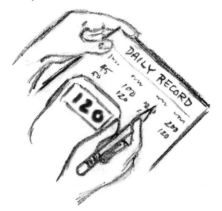

Blood Glucose Monitoring

Sometimes adjustments in your diabetes plan will be necessary to keep your blood glucose levels within a normal range. This is especially true if you are injecting insulin, which must be carefully balanced with food and exercise. But adjustments can't be made if you don't know what your blood glucose level is. This is where checking or self-monitoring of blood glucose comes into play.

Blood glucose measurements can be performed at any hospital or clinical laboratory and in many doctors' offices. Your caregiver will ask you to have your blood glucose checked regularly to see how well your gestational diabetes is responding to treatment.

At different times during the day, your blood glucose level will change. Sometimes it may be close to normal, but at other times it will be high or possibly low. Your health care team will ask you to check your blood yourself several times a day. This is very important, because knowing how your blood glucose varies throughout the day will allow your health care team to suggest an appropriate meal plan, and possibly an insulin regimen, to normalize your blood glucose.

Of course, the checks don't do any good if you don't pay attention to their results. Write down the results of each blood glucose check. These results will tell your health care practitioner how well your regimen is working to keep your blood glucose levels on target and whether or not changes are needed. You can use a notebook to record your results, or ask your health care team or pharmacist for a logbook. A sample blood glucose logbook is provided below.

How do you check your blood? There are two ways. In both, you first prick your finger with a special needle, called a lancet, to get a drop of blood. (It is usually less painful to prick on the side of

Sample Blood Glucose Logbook				
Date	Fasting blood glucose	1 hour after breakfast	1 hour after lunch	1 hour after dinner

your finger to the side of the fingernail rather than right on the end.) What you do next will depend on the type of blood glucose test you use. Ask a member of your health care team to walk you through the process you will be following.

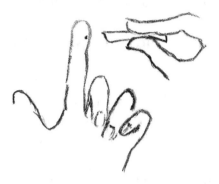

You place the drop of blood on a test strip (a chemically treated piece of paper or plastic) or in a blood glucose meter. A meter is a small computerized machine that "reads" your test strip. Your blood glucose level is displayed on a digital screen (like that of a pocket calculator). This is an accurate way to check your blood glucose level.

Women with gestational diabetes should check their blood glucose daily—four times a day for diabetes that is managed through meal planning and exercise and seven times a day if insulin is used in addition to a meal and exercise plan. It's a good idea to check it one hour after the beginning of each meal. You should also keep a daily record of what you ate at each meal. By looking at your logbook of test results, you and your health care team will be able to tailor your diabetes program to keep your blood glucose levels as close to normal as possible (below 90 mg/dl before meals and below 120 mg/dl one hour after meals).

A1C

Periodically, your health care provider may ask you to take a blood test called an A1C. This simple test tells what your average blood glucose level has been in the last two to three months. For people without diabetes, the reading is usually 5%, and during pregnancy you'll want to achieve that number or lower. If the value rises above 5%, your health care team will make adjustments to your treatment plan to help lower your blood glucose level.

Making Adjustments

As you work to manage your gestational diabetes, your health care team may ask you to make some adjustments—some major, some minor—in your meal plan or exercise routine or insulin regimen if you require one. While you are pregnant, your body undergoes changes that may affect your blood glucose level. Other factors, such as stress or unexpected physical activity, can also affect your blood glucose levels. You may have to make some adjustments to keep your blood glucose level on track.

If you take insulin, your health care provider will help you set up guidelines for making minor adjustments on your own, such as changes in the amount and type of snacks you'll need. For example, these guidelines will help you know what kind and how much of an extra snack you'll need before participating in an unexpected physical activity. However, if you are having a problem, such as high blood glucose every morning before breakfast, contact your health care team. Together, you can make adjustments in your entire regimen to better manage your blood glucose. Ask your doctor when you should notify him or her for such adjustments.

Again, recording the results of your blood glucose tests is very important. This information is vital to making adjustments in your diabetes regimen. As you and your health care team work together, you should be able to find a program that will keep you healthy.

More about Pregnancy

With the technology we have today, you can learn a lot about your baby even before it is born. Your health care team can check the baby's heart rate and the condition of the lungs, estimate the size and growth of a baby, and predict the sex of an infant before it is born. This technology is pretty amazing and can be comforting when you realize that it can increase your chances of having a healthy baby.

The tests we describe are used during all types of pregnancies, but they are particularly helpful in pregnant women with gestational diabetes. These tests help your health care team chart your baby's growth.

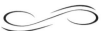

Chapter 8

Tests You Can Expect during Your Pregnancy

Tests to evaluate the growth and condition of your baby are known as antepartum tests. (Antepartum means before labor or childbirth.) The tests most often recommended for women with gestational diabetes are called fetal surveillance tests. They are usually given during the third trimester of pregnancy and often continue until delivery. Some of these tests measure your baby's growth. Others evaluate the baby's condition.

There are several tests that can be done. No method is clearly superior to the others. Different health care centers vary in their choice of tests. It is best to use the test (or tests) that a particular center is most familiar and comfortable with, since all methods are designed to provide similar information about your developing baby's health. Your health care team may request one or more of the following tests for you.

Ultrasound

Ultrasound tests use sound waves to outline and photograph organs—and developing babies—inside the human body. The picture that is taken is called a sonogram. This procedure has been used for about 40 years, and studies have not revealed any harmful effects to mothers or their babies.

If you've had this test performed before, you may remember that you were asked to drink lots of fluids before the test. To make sure that your bladder would be full, you were probably also asked not to urinate. Having your bladder full allows the person doing the test to make certain measurements more easily.

The procedure uses a machine with a monitor screen to produce the pictures. You simply lie back while a movable arm or probe (called a transducer) is gently glided across your abdomen. Ultrasound testing identifies the number of babies, their position in the uterus, and the outline and structure of their bodies.

Ultrasound can be safely performed throughout pregnancy. It can sometimes detect the sex of your baby, though sex determinations by ultrasound are not always accurate. It also helps in estimating how far along your pregnancy is.

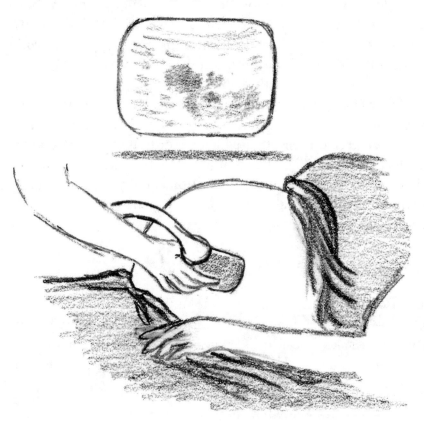

Because of the effects of gestational diabetes, your baby may be larger than average. Having several sonograms during the course of your pregnancy doesn't mean your baby is in any danger. Ultrasound is often performed at different times during a woman's pregnancy so that the health care practitioner can determine the baby's rate of growth.

Kick Counts

The movements or kicks that you feel from your baby are one important indicator of your baby's health. You may be asked to count the number of times you feel your baby move during a particular time period each day. Your doctor or nurse will explain how and when to do these counts. They will also explain how to recognize serious problems and when to alert your health care team. In general, when you detect a change in the pattern of your baby's movement, you should notify your health care team. They may want to do further testing.

Non-Stress Test

This test is used to determine the condition of your baby and the placenta. It is performed by attaching an electronic fetal monitor to your abdomen. The test measures changes in your baby's heart rate when he or she kicks, looking for the accelerations (speeding up) of your baby's heart rate at times of activity. These accelerations suggest that your baby is healthy. The test is painless and usually takes 30 to 45 minutes. It can be performed in your doctor's office or the hospital.

Contraction Stress Test

During a contraction stress test, as in the non-stress test, a fetal monitor is placed on your abdomen. The monitor prints out, on a strip of paper, your baby's heart rate response to a contraction of the uterus. It usually reflects how well the placenta transfers oxygen from you to your baby. You may be having frequent contractions, or your health care team may decide to start you on an IV and give you a hormone called Pitocin to start contractions, so that the response of the baby's heart rate to the stress of the contractions can be measured. This test can help to indicate the health of your baby and the placenta.

Biophysical Profile

In this test, ultrasound is used to evaluate your baby's movement, body tone, breathing, and the amount of amniotic fluid surrounding your baby.

Amniocentesis

Amniocentesis is performed by taking a sample of fluid from the amniotic sac (bag of waters) that surrounds the baby. This test can be performed in a doctor's office or hospital.

Ultrasound is used to find the baby and the best "pocket" of fluid. A needle is then inserted through the mother's abdomen to remove a small amount (usually less than an ounce) of the fluid. Either the fluid itself or the cells shed by the fetus into the fluid can then be studied.

In early pregnancy, the cells in the amniotic fluid can be analyzed for genetic abnormalities, such as Down's syndrome. In later pregnancy, amniocentesis can help determine if the baby's lungs are mature enough for the newborn to breathe on its own. This is important, because it is sometimes necessary to deliver the baby early by inducing labor or performing a cesarean delivery.

Chapter 9

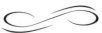

Labor and Delivery and Follow-Up

After examining your health and that of your baby and determining how well your pregnancy is progressing, your health care team will decide the best time and mode of delivery for both you and your baby. There are a variety of factors that will help your health care team decide the safest time and method to deliver your baby.

They'll study your baby's size and movements, his or her heart rate pattern, and the amount of amniotic fluid in the uterus. In some cases, a small amount of fluid will be withdrawn (see "Amniocentesis," page 58). This procedure will help determine whether your baby's lungs are mature and will help guide the timing of delivery.

Labor and Delivery

While you are in labor, your baby's heart rate and well-being will probably be monitored by a fetal monitor that is placed on the outside of your abdomen or by an internal monitor that is attached to the top of the baby's head after your water has broken. A soft, plastic catheter may also be placed inside your uterus to measure the strength and timing of your labor contractions. Your blood glucose level may be checked periodically during labor.

Most women with gestational diabetes have successful, complete pregnancies. For most, labor begins spontaneously, and they are able to deliver their babies vaginally (through the vagina). If your labor does not start on its own, it may be induced with a hormone called Pitocin. Pitocin speeds up labor by causing the muscles of the uterus to contract.

When a woman is unable to deliver her baby vaginally, she will have it delivered by an operation called a cesarean delivery (C-section). A C-section may be necessary if your baby is too large to fit safely through the birth canal. Other problems, such as the baby's position in the uterus, may also make a cesarean delivery necessary.

During a cesarean delivery, the baby is removed through an incision in the mother's abdomen and uterus. If you have a C-section, your recovery may be longer than if you delivered your baby vaginally. You will probably stay in the hospital for several days, and you will need 4 to 6 weeks to fully recover. Be sure to discuss both vaginal birth and cesarean delivery with your obstetrician months before your baby is born, so you will know what to expect.

In addition to the help your health care team can provide, many hospitals and other organizations offer childbirth education classes to help you prepare for the delivery of your baby. They teach you such things as what to expect during labor, techniques to improve delivery and to relieve pain during labor, and how to care for your baby after birth. If you're interested in such a class, ask a member of your health care team or check with your hospital about classes in your area.

Finally, we add this warning: Although some women want to give birth at home, home births are not recommended for women who have gestational diabetes because of the care needed to perform a successful delivery.

Follow-Up

Almost immediately after delivery, it's likely that your blood glucose level will return to normal. If you were injecting insulin to keep your blood glucose in the normal range, you will probably no longer need to do so. The extra hormones produced by the placenta that made your body resistant to the insulin you produced are now gone. However, women who have had gestational diabetes are at increased risk for developing type 2 diabetes in the future. For this reason, we recommend that you continue to monitor your blood glucose levels for one week after delivery. You should also have your blood glucose tested at your first postpartum checkup (a 2-hour glucose tolerance test with a 75-gram glucose load) and then yearly thereafter.

It's also possible that you will develop gestational diabetes again in future pregnancies, even if your blood glucose levels are normal between pregnancies. This is not the case for all women, but you should be checked for gestational diabetes when you become pregnant again and monitored closely.

Just because the gestational diabetes is gone does not mean you should let your guard down on healthy living. Protect yourself by eating nutritious foods, maintaining a healthy weight, and exercising regularly. Staying lean and fit after pregnancy will substantially lower your risk of developing type 2 diabetes in the future.

Breastfeeding

Nearly all women are encouraged to breastfeed their babies. Breast milk is healthy for the baby, and it contains antibodies to fight certain infections. Breast milk has other advantages, too—it is readily available, inexpensive, and convenient. In addition, breastfeeding will help you bond with your baby. Breastfeeding can also help you lose some of the weight you gained during pregnancy. It might even be a good way to lose any excess fat you had before you became pregnant. Breastfeeding has also been reported to help prevent type 1 diabetes from developing in the baby as it grows.

Most women lose between 12 and 15 pounds during the first week after giving birth. The total weight you gained during pregnancy should be gradually lost over a three-month period. If your health care team recommends that you lose weight, you can begin during the time you are breastfeeding. However, you should generally wait two to four weeks after your baby's birth before you begin to lose this weight.

While you are breastfeeding, it is important that you get the right amounts of calcium, fluids, and protein. Breast milk is amazingly constant in composition, but the quantity of milk changes depending on how much liquid you drink. If you reduce the amount of food that you eat, the quantity of your milk will also be reduced. You and your dietitian can discuss and plan your meals to fit your needs while you are breastfeeding. If you still have diabetes after delivery (this occurs in 10% of women with gestational diabetes), then your blood glucose levels need to be kept in the normal range to prevent too much glucose from entering into the milk from your bloodstream.

Although breastfeeding may be an excellent way to nourish your baby, you may be unable or unwilling to breastfeed. Some women are uncomfortable breastfeeding or have jobs that make breastfeeding on a regular schedule difficult. Others, because of health reasons, are unable to breastfeed. If you can't or don't want to breastfeed, don't feel guilty. Your baby can still get the nutrients he or she needs from a formula.

Birth Control

You may be wondering what a section on birth control is doing in a book about pregnancy. Maybe you think it's a little late to be talking about that now. But this book is not just for pregnant women. Birth control is an important topic both for women who are thinking about having a baby and for those who have already had a baby.

There are many birth control options on the market today, and it is important that you and your partner choose carefully. Some methods may work better and fit into your lifestyle more easily than others. Some are safer for you than others. Making an informed choice, which includes discussing birth control with your health care team, will help you select a method with a high success rate and fewer health risks.

Chapter 10

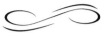

Making the Choice

Many women with diabetes are concerned about the safety of various methods of contraception and the advantages and disadvantages of each. One of the most important aspects of family planning is choosing the right method of birth control for you and your partner.

A number of different methods are available, and no one method is right for all individuals. You have special needs that may make one form of birth control better for you than another. The important factor in choosing any method is that it should be reliable and effective. Unfortunately, not all the methods available today offer the protection you need. You and your partner should discuss the options and find a birth control method that suits both of you. Make sure you also talk with your health care provider about the best choice for you.

Types of Birth Control

The Pill

Oral contraceptives, or birth control pills, are one of the most popular types of birth control. However, popularity doesn't mean the pill is the best choice for you. The advantage of birth control pills is their reliability. They are 99% effective when taken as directed.

"The pill" refers to a variety of oral contraceptives made from synthetic forms of two hormones involved in regulating the menstrual cycle, estrogen and progesterone. The synthetic form of progesterone is called progestin. A combination estrogen and progestin pill is slightly more effective than progestin alone (99% as compared to 98% success rate). The progestin-only pill can also cause irregular bleeding and weight gain.

In some instances, taking oral contraceptives can affect your blood glucose levels, even with today's with lower-dosage pills. If this is the case, your diabetes treatment program may need to be adjusted accordingly, or you and your partner will have to agree on other options. The pill may increase a woman's risk for heart disease or stroke and can cause a rise in blood fat levels (cholesterol, LDL, and triglyceride levels). It can also cause problems with circulation and clotting. In the newer pills, the lower dose of estrogen and progestin has decreased the risk for these problems.

For women who smoke, however, the risk for circulation and clotting problems is still quite high. Smoking causes the blood vessels to narrow, the walls of the vessels to thicken, and the blood to clot. That's why it is important for women to quit or reduce their smoking as much as possible. High A1C levels may also increase the chances of having blood-clotting problems.

If you choose to take oral contraceptives, it is important to have your A1C, blood fats, and blood pressure checked before and routinely after starting the pill. If you have high blood pressure or high blood fats (hyperlipidemia), you may need to use a different method of contraception. Taking the pill when you have high blood pressure can increase the chance that eye or kidney disease will get worse. If you are concerned, speak to your health care team.

Side effects from the pill, such as weight gain, irritability, breast pain, or breakthrough bleeding are more common with progestin-only pills. If you experience any discomfort with any oral contraceptive, it is important to discuss other options with your health care provider. For the best results, keep your blood glucose levels as close to normal as possible, take the pill as prescribed, and inform your health care provider when you have side effects.

Diaphragm

The diaphragm is a rubber cap that the woman lubricates with a spermicidal gel and fits into her vagina and over her cervix before intercourse. It acts as a barrier to prevent sperm from entering the uterus. The uterus is where eggs are fertilized by the sperm. For this reason, the diaphragm is called a barrier method of birth control. When used correctly, it can be up to 95% effective in preventing pregnancy.

Some women find a diaphragm awkward and difficult to use. And they fear it affects the spontaneity of lovemaking. Because the diaphragm can be inserted as much as an hour before intercourse, however, a little planning ahead will allow you to have some level of spontaneity. If you choose a diaphragm, your doctor will make sure it fits properly and will explain how to use it correctly. When women with diabetes use the diaphragm, they may have more yeast infections than woman without diabetes.

Condom

Another barrier method of birth control is the condom, a thin membrane sheath that fits over the penis. There are larger condoms for women that cover the outer labia and fit into the vagina. A condom can be used effectively by itself, but it is even more effective when combined with a sperm-killing foam or vaginal gel. Statistics show that when the condom and foam are used together, they are up to 85% effective in preventing pregnancy. The major problem with barrier methods of birth control, such as condoms, is that they require some planning for use. They must be used every time intercourse occurs, and they must be used correctly. If not, they won't be effective. Condoms also protect against the spread of sexually transmitted diseases (STDs).

Intrauterine Device (IUD)

An IUD is a small plastic device that is placed inside the uterus by a physician. It works by irritating the uterine wall, which makes it difficult for a fertilized egg to become implanted. In the past, some IUDs were suspected of causing pelvic infections or trauma to the uterine wall, but the newer IUDs are considered to be far less likely to do so. The IUD may be an attractive option for women who are not likely to have any more children and who have only one sexual partner (it does not protect against STDs). It is also an effective choice for women with diabetes because it does not affect blood glucose and blood fat levels. You should discuss with your health care provider any benefits or risks involved in using an IUD.

Rhythm Method

The oldest but by far the least effective method of birth control is the rhythm method. In general, it works by avoiding intercourse or using a barrier method during a woman's fertile phase—about 6 to 7 days before ovulation until 2 to 3 days after. For this method to work, you have to know exactly when you ovulate. Most women ovulate during the middle of their menstrual cycle. But cycles can be irregular, so it can be difficult to pinpoint the exact time of ovulation. The best, yet still inaccurate, method of determining when you ovulate is to measure your temperature. Body temperature rises slightly at the time of ovulation and remains elevated until your next period. To be as accurate as possible, you need to check your temperature daily in the early morning before you get out of bed. Since it is possible for pregnancy to occur 6 days before this rise in temperature, you must be diligent in measuring and recording your temperature patterns. You should not rely on this method if you have irregular periods or irregular body temperature patterns. The rhythm method does not protect against STDs.

Gestational Diabetes: What to Expect

Depo-Provera

Depo-Provera, a progesterone-like hormone, is given as an injection that prevents pregnancy for 12 weeks. This method has the advantage of being safe for use while breastfeeding (starting six weeks after delivery). However, Depo-Provera is not recommended for women who have had gestational diabetes.

Sterilization

Sterilization refers to either female tubal ligation ("tying the tubes") or male vasectomy. Both are simple surgical procedures that are permanent methods of sterilization.

After Your Baby Is Born

Finally, while we are on the subject of birth control, you may be wondering how soon after giving birth you can have intercourse. Unfortunately, there are no absolute answers to this question. It is probably a good idea to wait at least three or four weeks to give the muscles in the walls of your vagina time to strengthen. And if you have had an episiotomy, it will need time to heal. (An episiotomy is an incision made between the vagina and anus to help keep that area from tearing during the vaginal birth of your baby.) Check with your doctor to see how long he or she suggests you wait.

Remember that you can become pregnant soon after you give birth. Even if you have not had a menstrual period, you still may ovulate. Breastfeeding your baby will not prevent you from becoming pregnant.

Choosing birth control is a personal matter—the decision is up to you. But be sure to discuss the different types of birth control with your health care provider. The more information you have, the more likely you are to make the decision that is best for you.

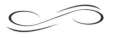

Conclusion

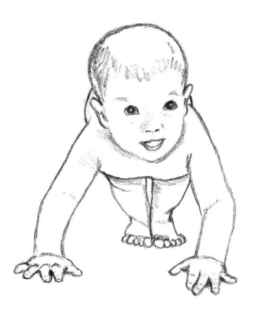

This book contains a lot of information, and some of what you read may seem overwhelming. Remember that your health care team is there to help you overcome any difficulties you may have. Your team will answer your questions and help you create a program, like those discussed in this book, to fit your needs and to work toward keeping your blood glucose levels within a normal range.

If you find yourself feeling frustrated or discouraged, you might try focusing on the end result of all your hard work—a happy, healthy, beautiful baby.

Appendix: Meal Planning

When you have gestational diabetes, you need to eat enough to stay healthy and to help your baby grow, but you should not eat too much. Having your own meal plan can help you make appropriate food choices. Make an appointment with a registered dietitian as soon as possible to create your meal plan. You can use the plans in this book to get started, but make sure that you check with your doctor or other health care practitioner first.

The sample meal plans in this book provide balanced meals, including appropriate amounts of carbohydrate, protein, and fat, for you and your baby. They also use the exchange system, which divides food into six groups or "exchange lists": starches or breads, fruit, milk, vegetables, meat or meat substitutes, and fat. You can "exchange" any food on one list for any other food on the same list. Ask your health care provider for a copy of the exchange lists, or contact the American Diabetes Association (1-800-DIABETES).

Sample 1,800-calorie, 2,000-calorie, and 2,200-calorie meal plans are provided on pages 76–87. You can use the body mass index (BMI) and weight classification charts to determine how many calories you need each day. There are two sample meal plans for each calorie level—one with milk and one without it. Although it is better if you can use the meal plan with milk, some people just do not like or cannot tolerate milk. If you do not drink milk, ask your doctor or dietitian about calcium supplements.

Daily Calorie Requirements

How do you know how many calories you need each day during your pregnancy? You can use the body mass index chart below to find out. First, locate your BMI using your height in inches and your weight before pregnancy.

BMI	19	20	21	22	23	24	25	26	27	28	29	30	31	32	33	34	35
Height (inches)	Body Weight (pounds)																
58	91	96	100	105	110	115	119	124	129	134	138	143	148	153	158	162	167
59	94	99	104	109	114	119	124	128	133	138	143	148	153	158	163	168	173
60	97	102	107	112	118	123	128	133	138	143	148	153	158	163	168	174	179
61	100	106	111	116	122	127	132	137	143	148	153	158	164	169	174	180	185
62	104	109	115	120	126	131	136	142	147	153	158	164	169	175	180	186	191
63	107	113	118	124	130	135	141	146	152	158	163	169	175	180	186	191	197
64	110	116	122	128	134	140	145	151	157	163	169	174	180	186	192	197	204
65	114	120	126	132	138	144	150	156	162	168	174	180	186	192	198	204	210
66	118	124	130	136	142	148	155	161	167	173	179	186	192	198	204	210	216
67	121	127	134	140	146	153	159	166	172	178	185	191	198	204	211	217	223
68	125	131	138	144	151	158	164	171	177	184	190	197	203	210	216	223	230
69	128	135	142	149	155	162	169	176	182	189	196	203	209	216	223	230	236
70	132	139	146	153	160	167	174	181	188	195	202	209	216	222	229	236	243
71	136	143	150	157	165	172	179	186	193	200	208	215	222	229	236	243	250
72	140	147	154	162	169	177	184	191	199	206	213	221	228	235	242	250	258
73	144	151	159	166	174	182	189	197	204	212	219	227	235	242	250	257	265
74	148	155	163	171	179	186	194	202	210	218	225	233	241	249	256	264	272
75	152	160	168	176	184	192	200	208	216	224	232	240	248	256	264	272	279

Source: National Heart, Lung, and Blood Institute

Gestational Diabetes: What to Expect

Now that you know your BMI, use the weight classification chart below to determine the number of calories per kilogram you need.

BMI	Weight Classification	Calories per Kilogram
Less than 20	Underweight	36–40
20–24	Normal weight	30
25–29	Overweight	24
30 or more	Obese	12–18

Next, convert your weight from pounds to kilograms by dividing your prepregnancy weight by 2.2. Multiply the result by the number in the calories per kilogram column for your weight classification.

This number will give you a good idea of how many calories you need each day. You can use the sample menus on the following pages to help you plan your meals. Keep in mind that all pregnant women need at least 1,800 calories a day.

Here is an example: Mary is 5 feet, 4 inches tall, and she weighed 164 pounds before she became pregnant. She converts her height to 64 inches (5 feet is 60 inches, plus 4 more equals 64) and looks at the BMI chart to find her BMI, which is between 28 and 29. She reads the weight classification chart, which tells her that a BMI of 28 to 29 is considered overweight. Mary sees that she needs to eat 24 calories per kilogram during her pregnancy. A kilogram is 2.2 pounds, so Mary divides her weight in pounds by 2.2 to get her kilogram weight. The result is 74.5 kilograms. Since she is overweight, a starting point for the number of calories she needs is 24 calories per kilogram. Mary multiplies 74.5 times 24 and gets 1,788 calories. Since Mary knows not go below 1,800 calories a day while she is pregnant, she chooses one of the 1,800-calorie meal plans as her starting point.

1,800-Calorie Meal Plan with Milk
Sample Meal 1: 45% Carbohydrate, 22% Protein, 33% Fat

		Exchanges	Carb (g)	Protein (g)	Fat (g)	Calories
Breakfast	1/2 cup cooked oatmeal	1 starch	13	3	1	73
	1 cup skim milk	1 fat-free milk	12	8	0	83
	1 hard-boiled egg	1 medium-fat meat	0	6	5	74
	1 tsp tub margarine	1 fat	0	0	4	34
	Breakfast Totals:		**25**	**17**	**10**	**264**
Snack	1 small roll	1 starch	14	2	2	85
	1 cup raw tomatoes	1 vegetable	7	2	0	32
	1 tsp tub margarine	1 fat	0	0	4	34
	Snack Totals:		**21**	**4**	**6**	**151**
Lunch	2 slices pumpernickel bread	2 starch	30	6	2	160
	1 cup skim milk	1 fat-free milk	12	8	0	83
	1/2 cup cooked broccoli	1 vegetable	4	2	0	22
	2 oz white meat chicken	2 very lean meat	0	18	2	93
	2 tsp mayonnaise	2 fat	0	0	7	66
	20 peanuts	2 fat	4	5	10	118
	Lunch Totals:		**50**	**39**	**21**	**542**
Snack	1 kiwi	1 fruit	13	1	0	56
	1 cup raw carrots	1 vegetable	12	1	0	50
	1 Tbsp salad dressing dip	1 fat	3	0	6	67
	Snack Totals:		**28**	**2**	**6**	**173**
Dinner	1/2 cup corn	1 starch	15	2	1	66
	1 1/4 cup strawberries	1 fruit	17	1	0	65
	1 cup skim milk	1 fat-free milk	12	8	0	83
	1/2 cup cooked kale	1 vegetable	4	1	0	18
	2 oz lean ground beef patty	1 medium-fat meat	0	14	9	137
	2 tsp tub margarine	2 fat	0	0	8	69
	Dinner Totals:		**48**	**26**	**18**	**438**
Snack	1/2 cup cereal (mix with yogurt)	1 starch	19	3	0	76
	3/4 cup plain nonfat yogurt	1 fat-free milk	14	9	0	90
	1 cup sliced raw zucchini	1 vegetable	4	1	0	18
	6 cashews	1 fat	3	1	4	52
	Snack Totals:		**40**	**14**	**4**	**236**
	DAILY TOTALS:		**212**	**102**	**65**	**1804**

1,800-Calorie Meal Plan with Milk
Sample Meal 2: 45% Carbohydrate, 22% Protein, 33% Fat

		Exchanges	Carb (g)	Protein (g)	Fat (g)	Calories
Breakfast	1 slice whole wheat toast	1 starch	13	3	1	69
	3/4 cup plain nonfat yogurt	1 fat-free milk	14	9	0	90
	1 oz ham, reheated to 165°F	1 lean meat	0	8	3	60
	1 1/2 tsp tub margarine	1 1/2 fat	0	0	6	51
	Breakfast Totals:		**27**	**20**	**10**	**270**
Snack	3 cups microwave popcorn	1 starch,1 fat	10	2	7	111
	1 cup raw celery	1 vegetable	4	1	0	17
	Snack Totals:		**14**	**3**	**7**	**128**
Lunch	1/3 cup brown rice	1 starch	15	2	1	71
	1/2 cup cooked pinto beans	1 starch, 1 very lean meat	22	7	0	116
	1 cup skim milk	1 fat-free milk	12	8	0	83
	1/2 cup cooked asparagus	1 vegetable	4	3	1	22
	1 oz reduced-fat Monterey Jack cheese	1 medium-fat meat	0	9	5	81
	1 tsp tub margarine	1 fat	0	0	4	34
	8 pecan halves	2 fat	2	1	8	80
	Lunch Totals:		**55**	**30**	**19**	**487**
Snack	12 sweet cherries	1 fruit	14	1	1	59
	1 cup mixed raw vegetables	1 vegetable	5	2	0	26
	1 Tbsp salad dressing	1 fat	3	0	6	67
	Snack Totals:		**22**	**3**	**7**	**152**
Dinner	1/2 cup boiled potatoes	1 starch	17	1	0	73
	1 cup cantaloupe cubes	1 fruit	13	1	0	56
	1 cup skim milk	1 fat-free milk	12	8	0	83
	2 cups mixed salad greens	1 vegetable	3	1	0	15
	2 oz roast lamb	2 medium-fat meat	0	15	8	132
	1 Tbsp sesame seeds, on salad	1 fat	2	2	5	52
	1 tsp olive oil, on salad	1 fat	0	0	5	40
	1 tsp vinegar, on salad	free food	0	0	0	0
	Dinner Totals:		**47**	**28**	**18**	**451**
Snack	2 inch cube of corn bread	1 starch, 1 fat	25	4	4	152
	1 cup skim milk	1 fat-free milk	12	8	0	83
	1 cup sliced green pepper	1 vegetable	4	1	0	18
	Snack Totals:		**41**	**13**	**4**	**253**
	DAILY TOTALS:		**206**	**97**	**65**	**1741**

1,800-Calorie Meal Plan without Milk
Sample Meal 1: 44% Carbohydrate, 21% Protein, 35% Fat

		Exchanges	Carb (g)	Protein (g)	Fat (g)	Calories
Breakfast	1 cup cooked oatmeal	2 starch	25	6	2	145
	2 hard-boiled eggs	2 medium-fat meat	1	13	10	147
	1 tsp tub margarine	1 fat	0	0	4	34
	Breakfast Totals:		**26**	**19**	**16**	**326**
Snack	3/4 oz pretzels	1 starch	17	2	1	80
	1 cup raw tomatoes	1 vegetable	7	2	0	32
	Snack Totals:		**24**	**4**	**1**	**112**
Lunch	2 slices pumpernickel bread	2 starch	30	6	2	160
	1 cup cooked broccoli	2 vegetable	8	5	1	44
	2 oz white meat chicken	2 very lean meat	0	18	2	93
	2 tsp mayonnaise	2 fat	0	0	7	66
	10 peanuts	1 fat	2	2	5	59
	Lunch Totals:		**40**	**31**	**17**	**422**
Snack	1/2 English muffin	1 starch	13	2	1	67
	1 kiwi	1 fruit	13	1	0	56
	1 cup raw carrots	1 vegetable	12	1	0	50
	Snack Totals:		**38**	**4**	**1**	**173**
Dinner	1/2 cup corn	1 starch	15	2	1	66
	1 1/4 cup strawberries	1 fruit	17	1	0	65
	1 cup cooked kale	2 vegetable	7	2	1	36
	3 oz lean ground beef patty	3 medium-fat meat	0	20	14	205
	2 tsp canola oil	2 fat	0	0	9	80
	Dinner Totals:		**39**	**25**	**25**	**452**
Snack	1/2 cup cereal	1 starch	19	3	0	76
	4 oz apple	1 fruit	15	0	0	55
	1 oz cheddar cheese	1 high-fat meat	0	7	9	114
	3 cashews	1/2 fat	1	1	2	26
	Snack Totals:		**35**	**11**	**11**	**271**
	DAILY TOTALS:		**202**	**94**	**71**	**1756**

1,800-Calorie Meal Plan without Milk
Sample Meal 2: 45% Carbohydrate, 21% Protein, 34% Fat

		Exchanges	Carb (g)	Protein (g)	Fat (g)	Calories
Breakfast	2 slices whole wheat toast	2 starch	26	5	2	138
	2 oz ham, reheated to 165°F	2 lean meat	0	17	5	120
	1 tsp tub margarine	1 fat	0	0	4	34
	4 walnut halves	1 fat	1	1	5	52
	Breakfast Totals:		**27**	**23**	**16**	**344**
Snack	1 slice raisin bread	1 starch	14	2	1	71
	1/2 cup raw peppers	1/2 vegetable	2	0	0	9
	1/2 cup raw cauliflower	1/2 vegetable	3	1	0	13
	Snack Totals:		**19**	**3**	**1**	**93**
Lunch	1/3 cup brown rice	1 starch	15	2	1	71
	1/2 cup cooked pinto beans	1 starch, 1 very lean meat	22	7	0	116
	1 cup cooked asparagus	2 vegetable	8	5	1	44
	1 oz reduced-fat Monterey Jack cheese	1 medium-fat meat	0	9	5	81
	1 tsp tub margarine	1 fat	0	0	4	34
	4 walnut halves	1 fat	1	1	5	52
	Lunch Totals:		**46**	**24**	**16**	**398**
Snack	8 animal crackers	1 starch	15	1	3	89
	1 cup cubed papaya	1 fruit	14	1	0	55
	1 cup raw celery	1 vegetable	4	1	0	17
	Snack Totals:		**33**	**3**	**3**	**161**
Dinner	1/2 cup mashed potatoes	1 starch	19	2	0	85
	1 cup cantaloupe cubes	1 fruit	13	1	0	56
	1 cup cooked green beans	2 vegetable	10	2	0	44
	3 oz roast lamb	3 medium-fat meat	0	22	11	198
	1 tsp tub margarine	1 fat	0	0	4	34
	6 almonds	1 fat	2	2	4	48
	Dinner Totals:		**44**	**29**	**19**	**465**
Snack	2 inch cube of corn bread	1 starch, 1 fat	25	4	4	152
	3/4 cup blackberries	1 fruit	14	1	0	56
	1 oz reduced-fat cheddar cheese	1 medium-fat meat	1	7	6	80
	Snack Totals:		**40**	**12**	**10**	**288**
	DAILY TOTALS:		**209**	**94**	**65**	**1749**

2,000-Calorie Meal Plan with Milk
Sample Meal 1: 40% Carbohydrate, 23% Protein, 37% Fat

		Exchanges	Carb (g)	Protein (g)	Fat (g)	Calories
Breakfast	1/2 cup cooked oatmeal	1 starch	13	3	1	73
	1 cup skim milk	1 fat-free milk	12	8	0	83
	2 hard-boiled eggs	2 medium-fat meat	1	13	10	147
	2 tsp tub margarine	2 fat	0	0	8	69
	Breakfast Totals:		**26**	**24**	**19**	**372**
Snack	3/4 oz pretzels	1 starch	17	2	1	80
	10 peanuts	1 fat	2	2	5	59
	Snack Totals:		**19**	**4**	**6**	**139**
Lunch	2 slices pumpernickel bread	2 starch	30	6	2	160
	17 small grapes	1 fruit	15	1	0	60
	1 cup skim milk	1 fat-free milk	12	8	0	83
	1/2 cup cooked broccoli	1 vegetable	4	2	0	22
	2 oz white meat chicken	2 very lean meat	0	18	2	93
	2 tsp mayonnaise	2 fat	0	0	7	66
	20 peanuts	2 fat	4	5	10	118
	Lunch Totals:		**65**	**40**	**21**	**602**
Snack	1/4 large bagel	1 starch	15	3	0	78
	1 small apple	1 fruit	15	0	0	55
	1 tsp tub margarine	1 fat	0	0	4	34
	Snack Totals:		**30**	**3**	**4**	**167**
Dinner	1/2 cup corn	1 starch	15	2	1	66
	1 cup skim milk	1 fat-free milk	12	8	0	83
	1 cup cooked kale	2 vegetable	7	2	1	36
	3 oz lean ground beef patty	3 medium-fat meat	0	20	14	205
	2 tsp tub margarine	2 fat	0	0	8	69
	Dinner Totals:		**34**	**32**	**24**	**459**
Snack	1 1/4 cup strawberries	1 fruit	17	1	0	65
	3/4 cup plain nonfat yogurt	1 fat-free milk	14	9	0	90
	1 oz cheddar cheese	1 high-fat meat	0	7	9	114
	3 cashews	1/2 fat	1	1	2	26
	Snack Totals:		**32**	**18**	**11**	**295**
	DAILY TOTALS:		**206**	**121**	**85**	**2034**

2,000-Calorie Meal Plan with Milk
Sample Meal 2: 43% Carbohydrate, 23% Protein, 34% Fat

		Exchanges	Carb (g)	Protein (g)	Fat (g)	Calories
Breakfast	1 slice whole wheat toast	1 starch	13	3	1	69
	3/4 cup plain nonfat yogurt	1 fat-free milk	14	9	0	90
	2 oz ham, reheated to 165°F	2 lean meat	0	17	5	120
	2 tsp tub margarine	2 fat	0	0	8	69
	4 walnut halves	1 fat	1	1	5	52
	Breakfast Totals:		**28**	**30**	**19**	**400**
Snack	1 slice raisin bread	1 starch	14	2	1	71
	1 tsp tub margarine	1 fat	0	0	4	34
	Snack Totals:		**14**	**2**	**5**	**105**
Lunch	1/3 cup white rice	1 starch	15	1	0	68
	1/2 cup cooked pinto beans	1 starch, 1 very lean meat	22	7	0	116
	17 small grapes	1 fruit	15	1	0	60
	1 cup skim milk	1 fat-free milk	12	8	0	83
	1/2 cup cooked asparagus	1 vegetable	4	2	0	22
	1 oz part-skim mozzarella cheese	1 medium-fat meat	1	7	4	72
	1 tsp tub margarine	1 fat	0	0	4	34
	8 pecan halves	2 fat	2	1	8	80
	Lunch Totals:		**71**	**27**	**16**	**535**
Snack	2 inch cube of corn bread	1 starch, 1 fat	25	4	4	152
	12 sweet cherries	1 fruit	14	1	1	59
	Snack Totals:		**39**	**5**	**5**	**211**
Dinner	1/2 cup mashed potatoes	1 starch	19	2	0	85
	1 cup skim milk	1 fat-free milk	12	8	0	83
	1 cup cooked green beans	2 vegetable	10	2	0	44
	3 oz roast lamb	3 medium-fat meat	0	22	11	198
	2 tsp tub margarine	2 fat	0	0	8	69
	Dinner Totals:		**41**	**34**	**19**	**479**
Snack	1 cup cantaloupe	1 fruit	13	1	0	56
	1 cup skim milk	1 fat-free milk	12	8	0	83
	1/4 cup nonfat cottage cheese	1 very lean meat	3	7	0	40
	12 almonds	2 fat	3	4	8	96
	Snack Totals:		**31**	**20**	**8**	**275**
	DAILY TOTALS:		**224**	**118**	**72**	**2005**

2,000-Calorie Meal Plan without Milk
Sample Meal 1: 42% Carbohydrate, 23% Protein, 35% Fat

		Exchanges	Carb (g)	Protein (g)	Fat (g)	Calories
Breakfast	1 cup cooked oatmeal	2 starch	25	6	2	145
	2 hard-boiled eggs	2 medium-fat meat	1	13	10	147
	1 tsp tub margarine	1 fat	0	0	4	34
	Breakfast Totals:		**26**	**19**	**16**	**326**
Snack	3/4 oz pretzels	1 starch	17	2	1	80
	10 peanuts	1 fat	2	2	5	59
	Snack Totals:		**19**	**4**	**6**	**139**
Lunch	2 slices pumpernickel bread	2 starch	30	6	2	160
	3/4 oz fat-free tortilla chips	1 starch	18	2	1	82
	1/2 cup cooked broccoli	1 vegetable	4	2	0	22
	3 oz white meat chicken	3 very lean meat	0	26	3	140
	3 tsp mayonnaise	3 fat	1	0	11	99
	10 peanuts	1 fat	2	2	5	59
	Lunch Totals:		**55**	**38**	**22**	**562**
Snack	1/2 English muffin	1 starch	13	2	1	67
	1 kiwi	1 fruit	13	1	0	56
	Snack Totals:		**26**	**3**	**1**	**123**
Dinner	1 cup corn	2 starch	30	4	2	133
	1 small roll	1 starch	14	2	2	85
	1 cup cooked kale	2 vegetable	7	2	1	36
	3 oz lean ground beef patty	3 medium-fat meat	0	20	14	205
	1 tsp tub margarine	1 fat	0	0	4	34
	Dinner Totals:		**51**	**28**	**23**	**493**
Snack	6 saltines	1 starch	13	2	2	78
	1 1/4 cup strawberries	1 fruit	17	1	0	65
	2 oz reduced-fat Monterey Jack cheese	2 medium-fat meat	0	18	10	162
	Snack Totals:		**30**	**21**	**12**	**305**
		DAILY TOTALS:	**207**	**113**	**80**	**1948**

2,000-Calorie Meal Plan without Milk
Sample Meal 2: 45% Carbohydrate, 20% Protein, 35% Fat

		Exchanges	Carb (g)	Protein (g)	Fat (g)	Calories
Breakfast	2 slices whole wheat toast	2 starch	26	5	2	138
	2 oz ham, reheated to 165°F	2 lean meat	0	17	5	120
	1 tsp tub margarine	1 fat	0	0	4	34
	4 walnut halves	1 fat	1	1	5	52
	Breakfast Totals:		**27**	**23**	**16**	**344**
Snack	1 slice raisin bread	1 starch	14	2	1	71
	1 1/2 Tbsp reduced-fat cream cheese	1 fat	1	2	5	54
	Snack Totals:		**15**	**4**	**6**	**125**
Lunch	2/3 cup white rice	2 starch	30	3	0	138
	1/2 cup cooked pinto beans	1 starch, 1 very lean meat	22	7	0	116
	1/2 cup cooked asparagus	1 vegetable	4	2	0	22
	2 oz part-skim mozzarella cheese	2 medium-fat meat	2	14	9	144
	20 peanuts	2 fat	4	5	10	118
	Lunch Totals:		**62**	**31**	**19**	**538**
Snack	8 animal crackers	1 starch	15	1	3	89
	1 cup cubed papaya	1 fruit	14	1	0	55
	Snack Totals:		**29**	**2**	**3**	**144**
Dinner	1 cup mashed potatoes	2 starch	37	4	1	170
	1/2 ear corn on the cob	1 starch	16	2	1	66
	1 cup cooked green beans	2 vegetable	10	2	0	44
	3 oz roast lamb	3 medium-fat meat	0	22	11	198
	1 tsp tub margarine	1 fat	0	0	4	34
	Dinner Totals:		**63**	**30**	**17**	**512**
Snack	1 reduced-fat waffle	1 starch	16	3	1	80
	3/4 cup blackberries	1 fruit	14	1	0	56
	2 pork sausage links	2 medium-fat meat	0	7	14	160
	Snack Totals:		**30**	**11**	**15**	**296**
	DAILY TOTALS:		**226**	**101**	**76**	**1959**

2,200-Calorie Meal Plan with Milk
Sample Meal 1: 41% Carbohydrate, 22% Protein, 37% Fat

		Exchanges	Carb (g)	Protein (g)	Fat (g)	Calories
Breakfast	1/2 cup cooked oatmeal	1 starch	13	3	1	73
	1 cup skim milk	1 fat-free milk	12	8	0	83
	2 hard-boiled eggs	2 medium-fat meat	1	13	10	147
	2 tsp tub margarine	2 fat	0	0	8	69
	Breakfast Totals:		**26**	**24**	**19**	**372**
Snack	3/4 oz pretzels	1 starch	17	2	1	80
	1 small apple	1 fruit	15	0	0	55
	10 peanuts	1 fat	2	2	5	59
	Snack Totals:		**34**	**4**	**6**	**194**
Lunch	2 slices pumpernickel bread	2 starch	30	6	2	160
	1 cup skim milk	1 fat-free milk	12	8	0	83
	1/2 cup cooked broccoli	1 vegetable	4	2	0	22
	2 oz white meat chicken	2 very lean meat	0	18	2	93
	2 tsp mayonnaise	2 fat	0	0	7	66
	30 peanuts	3 fat	7	7	15	177
	Lunch Totals:		**53**	**41**	**26**	**601**
Snack	1/2 English muffin	1 starch	13	2	1	67
	1 kiwi	1 fruit	13	1	0	56
	1 tsp tub margarine	1 fat	0	0	4	34
	Snack Totals:		**26**	**3**	**5**	**157**
Dinner	1/2 cup corn	1 starch	15	2	1	66
	1 small roll	1 starch	14	2	2	85
	1 1/4 cup strawberries	1 fruit	17	1	0	65
	1 cup skim milk	1 fat-free milk	12	8	0	83
	1/2 cup cooked kale	1 vegetable	4	1	0	18
	2 oz lean ground beef patty	2 medium-fat meat	0	14	9	137
	3 tsp tub margarine	3 fat	0	0	12	103
	Dinner Totals:		**62**	**28**	**24**	**557**
Snack	6 saltines	1 starch	13	2	2	78
	3/4 cup plain nonfat yogurt	1 fat-free milk	14	9	0	90
	1 oz reduced-fat Monterey Jack cheese	1 medium-fat meat	0	9	5	81
	6 cashews	1 fat	3	1	4	52
	Snack Totals:		**30**	**21**	**11**	**301**
	DAILY TOTALS:		**231**	**121**	**91**	**2182**

Gestational Diabetes: What to Expect

2,200-Calorie Meal Plan with Milk
Sample Meal 2: 44% Carbohydrate, 20% Protein, 36% Fat

		Exchanges	Carb (g)	Protein (g)	Fat (g)	Calories
Breakfast	1 slice whole wheat toast	1 starch	13	3	1	69
	3/4 cup plain nonfat yogurt	1 fat-free milk	14	9	0	90
	2 oz ham, reheated to 165°F	2 lean meat	0	17	5	120
	1 tsp tub margarine	1 fat	0	0	4	34
	8 pecan halves	1 fat	2	1	8	80
	Breakfast Totals:		**29**	**30**	**18**	**393**
Snack	3 cups microwave popcorn	1 starch, 1 fat	10	2	7	111
	1/2 large fresh pear	1 fruit	16	0	0	61
	Snack Totals:		**26**	**2**	**7**	**172**
Lunch	1/3 cup white rice	1 starch	15	1	0	68
	1/2 cup cooked pinto beans	1 starch, 1 very lean meat	22	7	0	116
	1 cup skim milk	1 fat-free milk	12	8	0	83
	1/2 cup cooked asparagus	1 vegetable	4	2	0	22
	1 oz reduced-fat cheddar cheese	1 medium-fat meat	1	7	6	80
	8 large black olives	1 fat	2	0	4	40
	1 tsp tub margarine	1 fat	0	0	4	34
	20 peanuts	2 fat	4	5	10	118
	Lunch Totals:		**60**	**30**	**24**	**561**
Snack	3 graham crackers	1 starch	16	1	2	89
	12 sweet cherries	1 fruit	14	1	1	59
	1/2 Tbsp peanut butter	1 fat	1	2	4	48
	Snack Totals:		**31**	**4**	**7**	**196**
Dinner	1 cup mashed potatoes	2 starch	37	4	1	170
	1 cup cubed cantaloupe	1 fruit	13	1	0	56
	1 cup skim milk	1 fat-free milk	12	8	0	83
	1/2 cup cooked green beans	1 vegetable	5	1	0	22
	2 oz roast lamb	2 medium-fat meat	0	15	8	132
	3 tsp tub margarine	3 fat	0	0	12	103
	Dinner Totals:		**67**	**29**	**21**	**566**
Snack	2 inch cube of corn bread	1 starch, 1 fat	25	4	4	152
	1 cup skim milk	1 fat-free milk	12	8	0	83
	1 sausage link	1 medium-fat meat	0	3	7	80
	Snack Totals:		**37**	**15**	**11**	**315**
	DAILY TOTALS:		**250**	**110**	**88**	**2203**

2,200-Calorie Meal Plan without Milk
Sample Meal 1: 40% Carbohydrate, 22% Protein, 38% Fat

		Exchanges	Carb (g)	Protein (g)	Fat (g)	Calories
Breakfast	1 cup cooked oatmeal	2 starch	25	6	2	145
	2 hard-boiled eggs	2 medium-fat meat	1	13	10	147
	1 tsp tub margarine	1 fat	0	0	4	34
	Breakfast Totals:		**26**	**19**	**16**	**326**
Snack	3/4 oz pretzels	1 starch	17	2	1	80
	1 small apple	1 fruit	15	0	0	55
	10 peanuts	1 fat	2	2	5	59
	Snack Totals:		**34**	**4**	**6**	**194**
Lunch	2 slices pumpernickel bread	2 starch	30	6	2	160
	3/4 oz fat-free tortilla chips	1 starch	18	2	1	82
	1/2 cup cooked broccoli	1 vegetable	4	2	0	22
	3 oz white meat chicken	3 very lean meat	0	26	3	140
	3 tsp mayonnaise	3 fat	1	0	11	99
	10 peanuts	1 fat	2	2	5	59
	Lunch Totals:		**55**	**38**	**22**	**562**
Snack	1/2 English muffin	1 starch	13	2	1	67
	1 kiwi	1 fruit	13	1	0	56
	1 tsp tub margarine	1 fat	0	0	4	34
	Snack Totals:		**26**	**3**	**5**	**157**
Dinner	1/2 cup corn	1 starch	15	2	1	69
	1 small roll	1 starch	14	2	2	85
	1 1/4 cup strawberries	1 fruit	17	1	0	65
	1/2 cup cooked kale	1 vegetable	4	1	0	18
	4 oz lean ground beef patty	4 medium-fat meat	0	27	18	274
	1 tsp tub margarine	1 fat	0	0	4	34
	Dinner Totals:		**50**	**33**	**25**	**542**
Snack	12 saltines	2 starch	26	3	4	156
	2 oz reduced-fat Monterey Jack cheese	2 medium-fat meat	0	18	10	162
	6 cashews	1 fat	3	1	4	52
	Snack Totals:		**29**	**22**	**18**	**370**
	DAILY TOTALS:		**220**	**119**	**92**	**2151**

Gestational Diabetes: What to Expect

2,200-Calorie Meal Plan without Milk
Sample Meal 2: 43% Carbohydrate, 21% Protein, 36% Fat

		Exchanges	Carb (g)	Protein (g)	Fat (g)	Calories
Breakfast	2 slices whole wheat toast	2 starch	26	5	2	138
	2 oz ham, reheated to 165°F	2 lean meat	0	17	5	120
	1 tsp tub margarine	1 fat	0	0	4	34
	4 pecan halves	1 fat	1	1	4	40
	Breakfast Totals:		**27**	**23**	**15**	**332**
Snack	1 slice raisin bread	1 starch	14	2	1	71
	1 cup cubed papaya	1 fruit	14	1	0	55
	1 tsp tub margarine	1 fat	0	0	4	34
	Snack Totals:		**28**	**3**	**5**	**160**
Lunch	2/3 cup white rice	2 starch	30	3	0	138
	1/2 cup cooked pinto beans	1 starch, 1 very lean meat	22	7	0	116
	1/2 cup cooked asparagus	1 vegetable	4	2	0	22
	2 oz reduced-fat Monterey Jack cheese	2 medium-fat meat	0	18	10	162
	20 peanuts	2 fat	4	5	10	118
	Lunch Totals:		**60**	**35**	**20**	**556**
Snack	8 animal crackers	1 starch	15	1	3	89
	1 cup cubed cantaloupe	1 fruit	13	1	0	56
	1/2 Tbsp peanut butter	1 fat	1	2	4	48
	Snack Totals:		**29**	**4**	**7**	**193**
Dinner	3/4 cup boiled potatoes	2 starch	34	3	0	146
	3/4 cup blackberries	1 fruit	14	1	0	56
	1/2 cup cooked green beans	1 vegetable	5	1	0	22
	4 oz roast lamb	4 medium-fat meat	0	30	15	264
	1 tsp tub margarine	1 fat	0	0	4	34
	Dinner Totals:		**53**	**35**	**19**	**522**
Snack	2 inch cube of corn bread	1 starch, 1 fat	25	4	4	152
	1/3 cup baked beans	1 starch	17	4	0	78
	2 sausage links	2 medium-fat meat	0	7	14	160
	Snack Totals:		**42**	**15**	**18**	**390**
	DAILY TOTALS:		**239**	**115**	**84**	**2153**

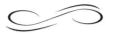

Glossary

Abruption (abruptio placentae): Separation of the placenta from the uterus while the fetus is in utero. It can be life threatening for the baby and requires emergency medical treatment.

American Diabetes Association (ADA): The nation's largest voluntary health organization dedicated to preventing and curing diabetes and to improving the well-being of all people affected by diabetes (for more information, see pages 101–102).

Amniocentesis: A procedure to take fluid out of the amniotic sac for tests.

Amniotic fluid: The fluid filling the amniotic sac.

Amniotic sac: Also known as the bag of waters. It is a fluid-filled sac that is attached to the placenta, in which the fetus develops.

Antepartum: Before delivery. For example, antepartum fetal monitoring means monitoring the fetus before delivery.

Bilirubin: A waste product of red blood cells that is excreted by the liver. Elevated bilirubin in the blood causes jaundice.

Biophysical profile: A test of fetal health that combines a sonogram with a non-stress test. The biophysical profile evaluates fetal movement, muscle tone, and breathing as well as the amount of amniotic fluid present.

Carbohydrates: Sugars and starches.

Cervix: The opening of the uterus into the vagina.

Cesarean delivery: Also called cesarean section or cesarean birth. An operation where an incision is made through the abdomen and uterus, through which the baby is removed. Cesarean delivery is usually performed if the baby cannot be delivered by the usual vaginal route.

Contraction Stress Test (CST): Also called an Oxytocin Challenge Test (OCT). In this test the mother's uterus is stimulated with oxytocin (Pitocin), a hormone from the pituitary gland, to cause a few mild contractions. During the contractions, the doctor monitors the fetus's heart rate, which can help to indicate the health of the baby and the placenta. These contractions are not enough to cause labor and usually stop as soon as the oxytocin is discontinued.

Diabetes mellitus: A group of diseases with one common factor: elevated blood glucose (sugar). Diabetes may be caused by a change or a combination of several changes in the body, including decreased secretion of insulin by the pancreas, high levels of hormones that act against insulin, or resistance of the body to insulin.

Diabetologist: A physician, usually an internist or endocrinologist, who specializes in the treatment of diabetes.

Dietetic: This term, which is often used in advertising, simply means one ingredient has been changed. It may mean fewer calories, less fat, less sugar, or less salt. It is not the same as diabetic, which usually refers to products containing less sugar or a different kind of sugar.

Dietitian: A health professional with special training in nutrition. A Registered Dietitian (RD) is a dietitian who has met the high standards of the American Dietetic Association and passed a national exam.

Endocrinologist: An internist specializing in endocrine and metabolic diseases, including diabetes mellitus.

Exercise: Any form of movement that burns energy.

Fat: Fats are the body's major storage system for energy. Dietary fats include margarine, shortening, oils, and butter.

Fetal monitor: A machine that monitors the heartbeat and activity of the fetus. One type (external) is placed on the mother's belly. The other (internal) is a small sensor placed on the baby's scalp during labor.

Fetal surveillance (or fetal monitoring): Tests to determine fetal well-being that are performed at varying times during the pregnancy.

Fetus: A term used for the developing baby while it is still in the mother's uterus.

Fiber: The indigestible portion of plant foods, such as the outer layer of grains or the woody part of many vegetables.

Gestation: Another word for pregnancy. May also refer to fetal development, such as the gestational (developmental) age of the fetus or newborn.

Gestational age: The age of the baby from the beginning of pregnancy. For example, after seven months of pregnancy, the baby's gestational age is 28 weeks.

Glucose: The body's main sugar, also called dextrose. Blood glucose is a measurement of the level of glucose that is in the blood.

Glucose challenge test: A screening test for gestational diabetes that is usually performed between the 24th and 28th week of pregnancy.

Glucose tolerance test: The definitive test to diagnose gestational diabetes. Usually done only if the glucose challenge test is abnormal. Blood glucose tests are taken each hour for three hours after drinking a liquid containing 100 grams (about 4 ounces by weight) of glucose.

Hormone: A chemical made by one cell or organ (gland) that is carried (usually in the bloodstream) to another cell or organ where it works.

Hyperglycemia: High blood glucose.

Hypoglycemia: Low blood glucose. Also called an insulin reaction.

Insulin: A hormone secreted by the pancreas. Insulin lowers the level of glucose in the blood. Insulin is also a medicine that is used to treat diabetes.

Intravenous: Given through a vein. Fluids and/or medications may be given intravenously—that is, directly into the bloodstream through a vein.

Jaundice: Yellowing of the skin and eyes caused by increased levels of bilirubin.

Ketone (acetone): An acid by-product of fat breakdown. Produced if there is not enough carbohydrate in the diet. Also produced if insulin levels are too low.

Labor: Muscular contractions in the uterus that squeeze down to deliver the baby.

Macrosomic: Describes a baby who is abnormally large for its developmental age.

Malformation: Birth defect.

Neonate: Newborn baby.

Neonatologist: A pediatrician specializing in the care of newborns.

Non-Stress Test (NST): A test of fetal well-being that monitors the baby's heartbeat and movements.

NPH or lente insulin: Intermediate-acting insulins.

Nurse educator: A nurse who has additional training and a special interest in diabetes education.

Obstetrician: A physician specializing in the care of pregnant women and delivering babies.

Oxytocin: A hormone from the pituitary gland that stimulates the uterus to contract. Small amounts of oxytocin (Pitocin) are used to stimulate mild contractions in the contraction stress test. Larger amounts are used to induce or stimulate labor.

Pancreas: An organ located in the abdomen behind the stomach and small intestine. The pancreas makes enzymes for digestion in the intestines and also secretes many hormones, including insulin, into the bloodstream.

Pediatrician: A physician who specializes in the care of infants and children.

Perinatal: Around the time of delivery.

Perinatologist: An obstetrician specializing in the care of complicated pregnancies. Also called a high-risk pregnancy specialist.

Pitocin: The brand name for oxytocin, a hormone used to stimulate contractions or induce labor.

Placenta: A specialized organ directly connected to both the mother's and the fetus's blood vessels. The placenta gets nutrients from the mother's blood for the fetus and secretes hormones necessary for normal pregnancy.

Postpartum: After delivery.

Prematurity: Birth of a baby before the full term of pregnancy is complete—usually used to describe any birth before 37 weeks of pregnancy.

Protein: Proteins, which are made up of amino acids, are the body's building blocks for muscle and bone. They are used for cell structure, hormones such as insulin, and other functions. Protein is also an essential part of the diet.

Regular insulin: Short-acting insulin.

Respiratory Distress Syndrome (RDS): A disease of the lungs causing breathing difficulty in the newborn baby. RDS is more common in premature babies and in the children of mothers with high blood glucose levels.

Starvation ketosis: A form of ketosis occurring when not enough carbohydrates are eaten.

Sterilization: A type of surgery undertaken to make a man or woman permanently unable to have children. This is usually done by an operation called a vasectomy (for men) or a tubal ligation (for women).

Trimester: One-third of the pregnancy. The first trimester includes weeks 1–12; the second, weeks 13–26; and the third, weeks 27–40.

Tubal ligation: An operation to cut the Fallopian tubes that carry the egg from the ovary to the uterus. As in a vasectomy, tubal ligation does not affect sexual function.

Type 1 diabetes: A type of diabetes that occurs when the pancreas can no longer secrete insulin. It is more common in young people but can occur at any age. Type 1 diabetes must be treated with insulin.

Type 2 diabetes: In type 2 diabetes, the pancreas may still secrete insulin, but the body is resistant to normal insulin levels. Type 2 diabetes may be treated with diet alone, with diet and exercise, or with a combination of diet, exercise, and oral drugs or insulin.

Ultrasound (sonogram): A sound wave picture of the fetus, placenta, and uterus. Ultrasound makes a picture of the area studied by bouncing sound waves off of it.

Uterus: Womb. The muscular organ in a woman's body that holds and nourishes the developing baby and in which the placenta develops.

Vaginal delivery: Delivery of the baby through the vagina.

Vasectomy: A minor operation to cut the tubes that carry sperm from the testicles to the penis. Vasectomy does not affect sex drive or the ability to have intercourse.

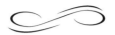

Index

About the American Diabetes Association

The American Diabetes Association is the nation's leading voluntary health organization supporting diabetes research, information, and advocacy. Its mission is to prevent and cure diabetes and to improve the lives of all people affected by diabetes. The American Diabetes Association is the leading publisher of comprehensive diabetes information. Its huge library of practical and authoritative books for people with diabetes covers every aspect of self-care—cooking and nutrition, fitness, weight control, medications, complications, emotional issues, and general self-care.

To order American Diabetes Association books: Call 1-800-232-6733 or log on to http://store.diabetes.org.

To join the American Diabetes Association: Call 1-800-806-7801 or log on to www.diabetes.org/membership.

For more information about diabetes or ADA programs and services: Call 1-800-342-2383. E-mail: AskADA@diabetes.org or log on to www.diabetes.org.

To locate an ADA/NCQA Recognized Provider of quality diabetes care in your area: www.ncqa.org/dprp

To find an ADA Recognized Education Program in your area: Call 1-800-342-2383. www.diabetes.org/for-health-professionals-and-scientists/recognition/edrecognition.jsp

To join the fight to increase funding for diabetes research, end discrimination, and improve insurance coverage: Call 1-800-342-2383. www.diabetes.org/advocacy-and-legalresources/advocacy.jsp

To find out how you can get involved with the programs in your community: Call 1-800-342-2383. See below for program Web addresses.

• *American Diabetes Month:* educational activities for people diagnosed with diabetes; occurs in November. www.diabetes.org/communityprograms-and-localevents/americandiabetesmonth.jsp
• *American Diabetes Alert:* annual public awareness campaign to find the undiagnosed; held the fourth Tuesday in March.

www.diabetes.org/communityprograms-and-localevents/ameri-candiabetesalert.jsp

- *The Diabetes Assistance & Resources Program (DAR):* diabetes awareness program targeted to the Latino community. www.diabetes.org/communityprograms-and-localevents/latinos.jsp
- *African American Program:* diabetes awareness program targeted to the African American community. www.diabetes.org/communityprograms-and-localevents/africanamericans.jsp
- *Awakening the Spirit: Pathways to Diabetes Prevention & Control:* diabetes awareness program targeted to the Native American community. www.diabetes.org/communityprograms-and-localevents/nativeamericans.jsp

To find out about an important research project regarding type 2 diabetes: www.diabetes.org/diabetes-research/research-home.jsp

To obtain information on making a planned gift or charitable bequest: Call 1-888-700-7029. www.wpg.cc/stl/CDA/homepage/1,1006,509,00.html

To make a donation or memorial contribution: Call 1-800-342-2383. www.diabetes.org/support-the-cause/make-a-donation.jsp